RELIGION AND SPIRITUALITY

RELIGION AND SPIRITUALITY FOR THE HEALTHCARE PROVIDER

RELIGION AND SPIRITUALITY

Additional books in this series can be found on Nova's website under the Series tab.

Additional e-books in this series can be found on Nova's website under the eBooks tab.

RELIGION AND SPIRITUALITY

RELIGION AND SPIRITUALITY FOR THE HEALTHCARE PROVIDER

BENJAMIN R. DOOLITTLE

NOVINKA
New York

Library of Congress Cataloging-in-Publication Data

ISBN: 978-1-63484-935-7

Published by Nova Science Publishers, Inc. † New York

To the hand in my hand
To the mermaids

Contents

PREFACE

There is compelling evidence that religious involvement and spiritual attitudes are beneficial to health. Religious involvement has been associated with increased lifespan, improved mood, improved coping with illness, and lower blood pressure and cholesterol. And yet, there is a "religiosity gap" between patients and their healthcare providers. Patients often have strong religious and spiritual attitudes that influence their perspective on health. Healthcare providers are often ill-equipped to address these issues.

Religion and Spirituality for the Healthcare Provider seeks to close that gap. Scholarly in scope, but approachable to all healthcare providers, Dr. Doolittle addresses the salient studies that explore the intersection of religion and health. He gives guidance about common challenges faced by healthcare providers: end of life issues, chronic illness, mental health, mindfulness and religious diversity. He also tackles controversies with the changing, complex role religion plays in modern society.

Dr. Doolittle is an internal medicine-pediatrics physician on the faculty of Yale Medical School. In addition, he is an ordained minister with active involvement in the urban church.

Chapter 1

WHY RELIGION MATTERS IN MEDICINE

Rosa[1] sits, head down, clutching her sides, rocking back and forth. She cries softly and moans over and over, "I am going to die. I am going to die. I know that I am going to die." She has just received news from a Department of Health Social Worker that she is HIV positive. She was then scheduled to see me that same day. I am a physician in my second year of residency, her doctor. Fortunately, my faculty has the expertise to supervise my care. With wonderful patient support services, excellent mentorship from faculty, and an earnest doctor-patient relationship, Rosa starts her HIV medications. Over time, her infection becomes well controlled, with an undetectable viral load and a robust improvement in her immune markers. More than that, she develops a positive outlook on life and finds a church home where she participates with increased enthusiasm.

Several years go by. I have joined the faculty of the clinic where I trained. Rosa is still my patient, always upbeat, still with an undetectable viral load and strong immune system. During one routine visit, I ask how she is tolerating her medications. She looks away, smiles wryly and say, "I stopped taking my medications about four months ago."

"Why?" I ask, miffed that she has stopped her life-saving treatment. She had been well controlled for many years and had no problem taking her medications before.

> "I believe that God has cured me of my HIV. I pray every day. I feel strong and healthy. I believe that God has cured me."

---

[1] To protect her identity, Rosa is not her real name.

That initial visit and the arc of her story over the years have spawned an abiding interest of the intersection of religion and health. In the spirit of full disclosure, I should have been more comfortable with her comments: I am an ordained minister as well as a physician. Throughout my medical career, I have had an active role in the ministry as a pastor of an urban church, usually in places that did not have other options but me. There was something very raw, very honest about Rosa's belief: she truly believed God cured her of her HIV. She was a reasonable woman, held a steady job, and was raising her young son. And yet, she had absolute confidence that God had cured her. What is more, her viral load was still undetectable, despite being off treatment for four months.

How did that happen, the movement from despair to certain faith? Why had she rejected her medications that, in my opinion, had saved her life? Had I failed her in some way? Did her medications remind her of her illness?

> "Rosa," I asked. "At church do you pray out loud with others?"
> "Yes, of course," she replied.
> "What do you pray for?" I asked.
> "For help. For strength. For healing. We pray all the time."
> "Would you mind if we prayed together?"
> Rosa smiles, "That would be wonderful!"

And so we did – the first time I ever prayed with a patient. I gathered our social worker and our nurse. They are good folks and understood what we were about. It seemed to make sense to pray in a group: we were all in this together. We prayed for hope, for continued good health, and for the commitment to stick together.

I did not want there to be an artificial separation between the church and the clinic. She felt comfortable praying with others. We had been doctor-and-patient for many years by then. We had gone through a lot together. And yet, even as a pastor, I felt off-balance about praying with a patient. As a pastor, I prayed with parishioners all the time. With a patient, in the clinic, it seemed out of place. Was it me? I called in the nurse and social worker much the way I would as if I were performing a pelvic exam. Prayer seems very personal, private, and intimate: I felt that I needed a chaperone.

We made a deal, Rosa and I. If you were not going to take your meds, fine. During those days, HIV physicians were kicking around the idea of a "drug holiday" to reduce the side effects of prolonged medication exposure. The plan would be to follow the T-cells and viral load, and restart the meds when things got dangerous. This practice has since been disproven, but at the time, it was within the realm of medical practice.

"Come and see me every three months, and let's make sure you are safe," was my suggestion.

With a confident smile, she agreed, as if she had secret knowledge of which I was not privy. She stuck to her end of the bargain. She came every few months. We checked her labs and made sure she felt okay. Surprisingly, her viral load remained undetectable for many years, and her T-cells were robust. I started to wonder if she were right. Did God cure her of her HIV?

This whole story colored by my own life as a religious person, a church pastor, with sermons to preach, and church events to plan. Why did I doubt so? Why was I so incredulous? Did I suspend my own faith while functioning as a physician? Over the years, we covered a lot of ground: medicines could be a gift from God. The church and the clinic need not be such dissimilar places. I was impressed by her faith, but also exasperated by what I perceived as her arrogance. What was it exactly? Was it denial of her illness masked as pride? And yet, she seemed so full of life.... We debated. We sparred. The years rolled by. Her T-cells were robust. Her viral load remained undetectable. Once I even repeated an HIV screening test to affirm that she was actually HIV positive. She declined the meds always with a wry smile and a sparkle in her eye. She had the gift of faith. She knew she would be okay, despite the imploring of her earnest young physician.

Our conversation subtly changed focus. "One of these days," I said. "You might be at risk for getting sick. Your T-cells are dropping and your viral load has begun to rise. By now, she was an expert in HIV medicine and knew exactly what that meant. When her T-cells dropped to 200 or so – the danger zone for serious opportunistic infections – my tone became more urgent. I attempted patience. I reasoned, disputed, cajoled and nothing worked. The months wore on.

One day, she acquiesced, "I need to be strong for God, for my church. I have much to do."

Three months after re-starting therapy, her T-cells had bounced back to a normal range. Her viral load was undetectable again after many years. And her counts continue to be so as of this writing. More importantly, she owns her therapy. Her HIV in some ways led her to a desperate faith that became real for her. Her faith then led her away from her HIV – or at least away from her HIV-related medical care. But now, she integrated the two worlds. There was no more debate or dissonance. She took her meds and got on with her life, serving God and raising her son.

Rosa's story exemplifies the complicated interplay between disease and belief, medicine and faith. She reconciled the two worlds - but it took years. This book is my attempt to make sense of Rosa's story and the larger issues of religion and medicine. I write from the perspective of a physician, curious about what makes my patients tick. I also write form the perspective of a Christian pastor, who has sweated Saturday night bouts of doubt and anxiety while preparing for the next day's sermon. I felt uncomfortable as an overtly religious, practicing minister; I can imagine how others might feel. This moment is precisely the reason why I wrote this book.

In modern medicine, there has been described a "religiosity gap" between health care providers and our patients (O'Connor & Vandenberg, 2005). Patients are much more likely to have an active religious life than their physicians (Koenig, 2000). Physicians tend to be selected with a talent for deductive reasoning and science. Thus, physicians have a natural predilection towards a biomedical illness model. Although medical schools are increasingly incorporating a more holistic, patient centered approach, the biomedical model predominates. We should note, without apology, that the biomedical, empirical, evidence-based model has produced widespread improvement in health and well-being for generations. It seems, though, that our greatest strength is also our weakness: it can be difficult to see beyond the empirical, rationalist, evidence-based training when treating and caring for patients.

It is important for clinicians to recognize our own limitations and biases when assessing our patients. This is not just a religious bias, of course, but also socio-economic class, race, education levels, and sexual identity. We are quick to judge; and in the realm of religion, we clinicians tend to judge negatively. We are quick also to assign pathology when, in fact, we are witnessing only cultural norm. We are quick to overlook the importance of religion – perhaps transferring our own predilection for the small role of religion in our own lives. In judging prematurely or overlooking altogether the role of religion, we miss out on an important coping strategy and a beautiful aspect of our patients' lives. Recognizing our limitations and biases is key towards all of patient care and towards religion in particular. The practical approach to this to ask, "Is religion important to your life?" I wonder if perhaps we feel more uncomfortable about this question than we do asking about sexual behavior and drug use.

There are more comprehensive compilations in the literature that this book. Harold Koenig's tremendous *Handbook of Religion and Health*, which came out in a 2nd edition in 2012, is exhaustive (Koenig, King, & Carson, 2012). His leadership in this field is unparalleled with more than 40 books and more than 400 articles. With his mentorship and his expertise, he energizes this field like no other. Christina Pulchalski, from George Washington University, has elucidated these questions of religion and health from the perspective of a palliative care physician. There are many others – Pargament, Culrin, the Balbonis and on and on. Many programs have popped up at medical schools to provide a home for scholarly work and interdisciplinary conversation.

This book is different. I am a primary care physician and a church pastor. And so, my question is this: how does this literature help me care for my patients? What studies are relevant? What do I need to know? This book seeks to answer that question. More than that, I am an enthusiast of these questions and recognize their complexity. What studies have influenced my own perspective the most? This work is meant to be a guide to these questions for anyone who provides healthcare to patients. Since scholarly work is ever expanding and more comprehensive tests appear everywhere, my hope is to raise up the very best that the scholarship has to offer. Hopefully, I will do so in a manner approachable to all.

REFERENCES

Koenig, H., King, D., & Carson, V. B. (2012). *Handbook of religion and health*. Oxford, UK: Oxford university press.

Koenig, H. G. (2000). Religion and medicine I: historical background and reasons for separation. *The International Journal of Psychiatry in Medicine*, *30*(4), 385-398.

O'Connor, S., & Vandenberg, B. (2005). Psychosis or faith? Clinicians' assessment of religious beliefs. *Journal of Consulting and Clinical Psychology*, *73*(4), 610.

Chapter 2

CONTROVERSY AND CHALLENGE IN RELIGION AND HEALTH

There is a physician archetype that pervades common culture: one of the beleaguered, overworked, over-stressed physician who never seems to have enough time. There are studies that support this. A 2012 survey of more than 7,000 physicians reveals that 44% consider themselves burned out (Shanafelt et al., 2012). There is another dimension to the archetype of the busy physician: patient expectations. In one study, 362 videotaped primary care visits were analyzed. The median length of visit was 15.7 minutes, covering a median of 6 topics, an average of 2.6 minutes per topic (Tai-Seale, McGuire, & Zhang, 2007). Patients are sicker and providers have less time to deal with them. Of these problems, a significant number of patients in a primary care practice will have a mental health disorder. In one series of an urban family practice, 40% of patients met criteria for a mental health disorder (National Ambulatory Medical Survey, 2008). 52% of all mental health visits in the United States occur within the primary care arena, without input by psychiatry (Kessler, 2012). These emotional issues are often more time-consuming and emotionally demanding than straight-forward "medical" issues. Why is this happening? Are we getting better at diagnosing these problems, or are they genuinely on the rise?

I would like to challenge these prevailing archetypes of the beleaguered, burned out physician and the needy patient. I believe the vast majority of physicians deeply care and seek the best for their patients. Our concern is genuine, heartfelt, and personal. While medicine can be regarded as a business, most physicians truly care and seek to live a comfortable life where money is not the primary driver.

In medical school, I served a small inner-city congregation. I would often write my sermons at the nurses' station while on call. One day, my attending approached me and quipped, "Doctors are the priests for today." He went on to state that patients in our post-modern age now approach their physicians much as people would approach their clergy-person. Years later, I am not sure if he was belittling my role as a pastor, commenting about our post-modern society, or both. Over the years, as I reflect upon that moment, I believe that he is right. Patients bring their pain and worry to their provider, much like a congregant brings their pain and worry to their pastor. To the doctor, often the worry is manifest as physical symptoms - lethargy, headaches, chronic pain – or even overt depression or subtler dysthymia.

In another sense, this idea of "physicians as the priest for today" represents an opportunity for every physician. Spiritual and emotional health matters a great deal to our patients and greatly impacts their health, as this book will point out. If a physician can address these issues with patients explicitly, this presents an opportunity for more comprehensive healing and a better doctor-patient experience.

Throughout the Middle Ages and into the 18th century, the clergy were an important provider of healthcare – especially in rural areas. The clergy were often the most educated, the most literate, in the community. More than that, the local clergyman was trained in rudimentary medical practices to care for the community in body and soul. The recent division between the worlds of medicine and ministry occurred during the Age of Enlightenment, the 18th century, when reason trumped faith and empiricism trumped revelation as the tool to understand the world. In many ways, this was appropriate. With the rise of technology and the implementation of the empiric method, the body of medical knowledge became too vast for clergy to assume proficiency with a few courses.

To this day, there remains tension between the worlds of science and religion. In recent years, there has been considerable excitement about the "God particle" – the Higgs Boson - which solved so many mysteries within particle physics. But many scientists have made the jump from physics to theology. Laurence Kraus, a physicist from Arizona State University, quipped in the New York Times, "If we can describe the laws of nature back to the beginning of time without any supernatural shenanigans, it becomes clear that you don't need God." (Lisee, 2012) Richard Dawkins, Sam Harris, Christopher Hitches and other so-called "new atheists" critique religion as being responsible for widespread ignorance, wars, and much of the moral depravity of society. Dawkins wrote in his book, *The God Delusion*, "The take-home message is that we should blame religion itself, not religious extremism - as though that were some kind of terrible perversion of real, decent religion. Voltaire got it right long ago: 'Those who can make you believe absurdities can make you commit atrocities.' So did Bertrand Russell: 'Many people would sooner die than think. In fact they do." (Dawkins 2008) He writes elsewhere, "The God of the Old Testament is arguably the most unpleasant character in all fiction: jealous and proud of it; a petty, unjust, unforgiving control-freak; a vindictive, bloodthirsty ethnic cleanser; a misogynistic, homophobic, racist, infanticidal, genocidal, filicidal, pestilential, megalomaniacal, sadomasochistic, capriciously malevolent bully." (Dawkins, 2008) There is widespread support, or at least curiosity, of his work. Dawkins' *The God Delusion* was a New York Times #2 best seller.

The post-modern era has been particularly hostile towards religion. Indeed, it was almost trendy to predict the decline of religion – ever since TIME magazine declared that "God is dead" on the cover of their April 8th, 1966 edition. A position paper from the National Academy of Sciences reported, "Religion and science are mutually exclusive realms of thought whose presentation in the same context leads to misunderstanding of both scientific theory and religious belief." (Ward, 1995) Religious experience has also been labeled, "a psychotic episode" (Horton, 1974), and, "temporal lobe dysfunction" (Mandel, 1980).

But not all physicians have felt this way. Sir William Osler, the founder of the modern residency education system, wrote, "Nothing in life is more wonderful than faith – the one great moving force which we can neither weigh in the balance nor test in the crucible.... Mysterious, indefinable, known only by its effects, faith pours out an unfailing stream of energy while abating neither jot nor tittle of its potency" (Osler 1910).

My own conviction is that we have entered an age of extremism. Religious extremism seems to be on the rise. Christian fundamentalism is manifest in several political groups such as the Tea Party movement as well as Muslim fundamentalism in the Islamic State. In the same way, scientific extremism seems to be on the rise with the work of Dawkins and others.

What is the clinician to do? What does the evidence say? This book is my attempt to answer that very question. While most patients have some religious belief, this domain has only recently been explored in rigorous fashion. In one of the earliest and most important systematic reviews of four psychiatric journals between 1978-1982, only 2.5% of the articles included some measure of religion (Larson et al., 1986; Weaver et al., 1998, Shafranske, 1996). Between 1991-1995, that number was only 1.2% (Weaver 1998). Further, religion was explored using a simplistic single question about denomination or religiosity in 80% of the studies (Shafranske 1996).

As our society has become more pluralistic and secular, we have made a distinction between being "spiritual" and "religious." Indeed, a national survey found that about half of American adults (52%) rated themselves as religious *and* spiritual, 10% as spiritual only, 9% as religious only, and 29% as neither religious nor spiritual (Shahabi et al., 2002). In an increasingly secular society, it has become trendy to be "spiritual" but not "religious." "Religion" implies doctrinal, traditional beliefs, even old-fashioned ones. "Spiritual" refers to an individual's attempt to find meaning in life, connecting with the transcendent, and is often outside traditional or institutional boundaries (D'souza & George, 2006). "Spiritual" connotes free-thinking, open-minded, ethical. "Spirituality" implies an individual search for the divine.

Critics of this post-modern perspective would point out the religious views are communal whose truths have stood the test of time. Relational aspects of religious practice are important. "Spiritual," in turn, is egocentric. Critics might say that the lack of structure and discipline leaves a "spiritual" person adrift. Anything goes. And yet, in medicine, perhaps "spirituality" is a safer term – like asking a patient about "relations" when you mean "sexual intercourse." Both "spiritual" and "religious" are loaded terms, and may make a clinician uncomfortable – perhaps even more so than asking about sexual practices or drug use.

"Religion" comes from the Latin *religare* which means "to fasten," "to bind." A religion is the set of beliefs that a community holds to be true that concerns the nature and purpose of the universe. At its core, religion "binds" us, connects us, to God, to one another, to the world. "Spiritual" is derived from the Latin *spiritus* which pertains to breathing, respiring, living. "Spirituality" concerns the invisible powers that give life and animation. The opposite of "spiritual" is "physical." A spiritual person, then, concerns herself with the invisible forces that give life.

There is considerable disagreement between the meanings of the terms "religiosity" and "spirituality." Religion is thought to be an outward, formal, institutional expression of the sacred and divine. Religiosity is often measured by asking about the importance of religion, belief in God, frequency of attendance at religious services, or other group activities. Spirituality is defined as an internal, personal, and emotional expression of the sacred and is measured by exploring spiritual well-being, peace and comfort derived from faith and spiritual connectedness (Hill & Pargament 2003; Miller & Thoresen, 2003).

Several researchers argue against the bifurcation of religiosity and spirituality. Instead, they posit a model of "proximal" and "distal" qualities. Distal qualities are regarded as the external manifestations of religion: religious attendance and frequency of prayer. Proximal qualities – those qualities closer to the heart – are the positive or negative religious coping, community support, or sense of peace that one derives from religion. Taken together – the proximal and distal domains of religiosity and spirituality – these factors impact health outcomes (Pargament, Koenig, & Tarakeshwar, 2000; Pargament et al., 2001). Thus, "spiritual" and "religious" are quite different concepts – both in their etymology and in our own modern understanding. Even so, these terms are not exclusive. Spiritual people can be religious and vice-versa.

In the research setting, it is important that these terms are well defined (Powell, Shahabi, & Thoresen, 2003). In particular, "spiritual" is associated with positive outlook, balance, satisfaction, and peace. When studying mental health and emotional issues, measuring spirituality can merely be a measure of satisfaction with life or lack of depression. These variables may be tightly correlated, but they will not be giving useful information: they often merely ask the same type of questions using different validated scales. Spirituality, in the research world, is often a proxy for emotional wellness (Powell, Shahabi, & Thoresen, 2003).

In the 19th century, the philosopher William James wrote the *The Varieties of Religious Experience*. He articulated a more nuanced critique of religion compared to the more polemical Freud (James, 1902). He described how there is a difference between one's personal religious sensibilities and that of the institutional church. He connected one's individual experiences with "nervous instability" and abnormal psychological processes. These mystical, personal experiences extended from a primordial source. In contrast, the institutional church is the product of culture and external forces. He was among the first to articulate a difference between personal religiosity and communal participation. James believed that there were no true personal religious experiences. Rather, they were personal experiences interpreted within a religious context (James 1902).

Religion can be difficult to study because it is such a complicated construct. There are powerful community practices, deep, important personal practices, existential beliefs about the nature of God and the universe, and a moral behavioral norm. What aspects of religion really matter to health? Further, the intensity of religiosity can vary widely. A person might consider themselves "religious" and have a deep, rich personal devotion, but spotty attendance at worship services, and a middling moral code. Researchers have devised several scales in attempt to capture this complexity but with varying success. In surveying patients, there is often a trade-off between length and response. Longer survey instruments may capture more nuance of belief - but perhaps result in a lower response from study subjects. Shorter surveys gather the essential and may result in a higher yield, but may not discriminate the nuances of religious belief.

Some researchers maintain that religion and spirituality can never be accurately measured. The topic is too personal, too deep-seated, or too sensitive for a participant to respond honestly to a survey. Further, the topic is too nuanced, too complex, for a survey to capture true sentiment accurately. I disagree with this position. Certainly, no survey instrument can capture all the subtlety of religious belief, but many have been validated in the literature and used widely with success. Many other similarly complex constructs – such as culture for example – have successful survey instruments. Why should religious belief be any different? Further, we must try. We must try to understand religion and spirituality, for the simple reason that our patients are religious and spiritual.

Taking a Spiritual History

In medical school, we are taught the importance of the social history and its impact on illness. Who do you live with? Do you smoke? Do you drink? Are you sexually active? With whom? We recognize that it is not enough simply to ask about drug and alcohol use or sexual preferences. As Hippocrates is credited as saying, "It's far more important to know what person the disease has than what disease has the person." In recent years, an entire discipline has evolved that focuses on the doctor-patient relationship. There are national organizations, such as the American Academy on Communication in Healthcare and the Schwartz Center for Compassionate Healthcare, that researches and advocates for best methods in fostering a rich, compassionate doctor-patient relationship. We have become more sophisticated in our medical school curricula. Entire courses that focus on doctor-patient communication have become de rigueur.

And yet, I wonder if medical students feel more comfortable with asking about sexual practices and drug abuse than about religious belief. Perhaps it is the deeply personal nature of religious belief, or perhaps the unresolved questions that a provider may have – especially one steeped in the traditions of science and evidence-based medicine. Perhaps, in the rush of modern medicine, getting around to the spiritual history is simply too difficult. Sex and drugs have a direct impact upon health in a tangible way – infections, liver disease, and accelerated vascular disease. Religious sentiment is subtler and its direct impact on health may not be so obvious.

Interestingly, patients hope for their provider to ask about their spiritual lives. While medicine has become more technical, driven more by scientific evidence, our patients are asking for something more. In one classic study in a primary care setting, patients were asked if their religion was important to them. 51% of patients described themselves as religious. 90% believe that prayers may sometimes influence recovery. 45% believe that religious beliefs would influence their decision making if gravely ill. 66% of patients would want physicians to ask about their religious beliefs – and this includes those who claim no religious belief. Only 15% of patients recalled being asked about their spiritual or religious beliefs by a physician (Ehman et al., 1999). Perhaps most care providers will acknowledge the importance of a patient's spiritual life in their care. Most have little resources in how to address this aspect of their lives. There is a disconnect between our patients' needs and the providers attitudes.

There are several models that can guide a practitioner to explore spirituality and religion with patients. For a model to be useful, it must be easy to remember, brief, appropriate, patient-centered and validated in the literature. The FACT Spiritual History Tool is one such model that was developed for healthcare providers and uses the mnemonic FAITH (LaRocca-Pitts, 2009):

> F (Faith): What is your Faith or belief? Do you consider yourself a person of Faith or a spiritual person? What things do you believe that give your life meaning and purpose?
>
> A (Active, Available, Accessible): Are you currently Active in your faith community? Are you part of a religious or spiritual community? Is support for your faith Available to you? Do you have Access to what you need to Apply your faith (or your beliefs)? Is there a person or a group whose presence and support you value at a time like this?
>
> C (Coping, Comfort, Conflict, Concerns): How are you Coping with your medical situation? Is your faith (your beliefs) helping you Cope? How is your faith (your beliefs) providing Comfort in light of your diagnosis? Do any of your religious beliefs or spiritual practices Conflict with medical treatment? Are there any particular Concerns you have for us as your medical team?

T (Treatment): Based on the responses to these questions, the clinician now makes a judgment as to the appropriate Treatment.

Another model that is briefer than the FACT Spiritual History Tool was developed by Harold Koenig (Koenig, 2002). Koenig (2002) proposes the CSI-MEMO Spiritual History that has four questions:

1. Do your religious/spiritual beliefs provide Comfort, or are they a source of Stress?
2. Do you have spiritual beliefs that might Influence your medical decisions?
3. Are you a MEMber of a religious or spiritual community, and is it supportive to you?
4. Do you have any Other spiritual needs that you'd like someone to address?

There are several important features to these two models. First, these questions recognize that not every religious affiliation is supportive. Faith is always in evolution – especially during times of illness. Religious doctrine may offer positions counter to the belief of the patient in regards to end of life care, abortion, blood transfusions, cost of care, and on and on. Further, the local religious community may have nuanced cultural expectations that may cause strife. Religious belief is interwoven into all aspects of life. An old member at my church once quipped, "When church is at its best, there is nothing better. When church is at its worst, there is nothing worse." We are wise to ask about the positive and negative aspects of religious affiliation. Second, this model asks directly how religious belief might influence medical decision-making, which can be very helpful during times of acute illness and hospitalization.

Another model proposed by a consensus panel of the American College of Physicians suggests 4 questions that a provider might ask a patient (Lo & Snyder, 1999):

1. Is faith (religion, spirituality) important to you in this illness?
2. Has faith been important to you at other times in your life?
3. Do you have someone to talk to about religious matters?
4. Would you like to explore religious matters with someone?

The common theme to these three models is that we should ask. As a primary care provider, delving into the spiritual beliefs of our patients is part of richness of our profession. Our patients regard us as more than caretakers of their bodies, but of the whole person. Supporting a patient's belief system deepens the doctor-patient relationship. One might argue that it takes too much time and opens a line of conversation that simply does not fit into the 15-minute patient slot. And yet, in the on-going relationship with our patients, which often span many years, asking about their spiritual lives, at least once, can yield dividends. Patients who trust their doctors use fewer resources, require less time, and sue less often. More than that, inquiring about our patients' spiritual lives gives depth and understanding to the struggles of our patients. They become more human to us.

The other important aspect to inquiring about our patients' spiritual lives is to elicit the support of the faith community in their support and care. Our patients have abundant needs, beyond case management support, coordination of referrals, and visiting nurses. Encouraging our patients to build deeper ties with their faith community forges a stronger support system. Often our patients have tenuous relations with their faith community – especially among patients whose illnesses carry a strong social stigma such as HIV or addiction. Rekindling a healthy relationship with a faith community creates one more platform of support – and perhaps may alleviate some of the pressure of the primary care provider.

REFERENCES

D'souza, R., & George, K. (2006). Spirituality, religion and psychiatry: its application to clinical practice. *Australasian psychiatry*, *14*(4), 408-412.

Dawkins, R. (2008). *The god delusion*. Boston, MA: Houghton Mifflin Harcourt.

Ehman, J. W., Ott, B. B., Short, T. H., Ciampa, R. C., & Hansen-Flaschen, J. (1999). Do patients want physicians to inquire about their spiritual or religious beliefs if they become gravely ill? *ArcHIVes of Internal Medicine*, *159*(15), 1803-1806.

Hill, P. C., Pargament, K. I. (2003). Advances in the conceptualization and measurement of religion and spirituality: implications for physical and mental health research. *American Psychologist*, 58(1), 64 –74.

Horton, P. C. (1974). The Mystical Experience: Substance of an Illusion, *American Psychoanalytic Association Journal* 22:(2): 364-380.

James, W. (1902). *The varieties of religious experience: A study of human nature.* New York: Random House.

Kessler, R. C., Avenevoli, S., Costello, J., Green, J. G., Gruber, M. J., McLaughlin, K. A., ... & Merikangas, K. R. (2012). Severity of 12-month DSM-IV disorders in the national comorbidity survey replication adolescent supplement. *ArcHIVes of general psychiatry*, *69*(4), 381-389.

Koenig, H. G. (2002). An 83-year-old woman with chronic illness and strong religious beliefs. The Journal of the American Medical Association, 288(4), 487–493.

LaRocca-Pitts, M. A. (2009). FACT: Taking a spiritual history in a clinical setting. *Journal of health care chaplaincy*, *15*(1), 1-12.

Larson, D. B., Mansell, E., Pattison, M. D., Blazer, D. G., Omran, A. R., & Kaplan, B. H. (1986). Systematic Analysis of Research on Religious Variables. *American Journal of Psychiatry*, *1*(43), 329.

Lisee, C. (2012 July 13). "God particle" discover ignites debate over science and religion. *The Washington Post.* Retrieved February 1st, 2016 from https://www.washingtonpost.com/national/on-faith/god-particle-discovery-ignites-debate-over-science-and-religion/2012/07/13/gJQAOpaWiW_story.html.

Lo, B., Snyder, L. (1999). Discussing palliative care with patients. *Annals of Internal Medicine.* 130(9); 772-775.

Mandell, A. J. (1980). *Toward a psychobiology of transcendence: God in the brain* (pp. 379-464). New York: Springer.

Miller, W. R., & Thoresen, C. E. (2003). Spirituality, religion, and health: An emerging research field. *American psychologist, 58(1), 24.*

National Ambulatory Medical Survey 2008 Survey Tables; Center for Disease Control, Mental Health Work Group, 4770 Buford Hwy, NE MS K-51, Atlanta, Ga. 30341-3717.

Osler, W. (1910). The faith that heals. *British Medical Journal.* 1:1470-72.

Pargament, K. I., Koenig, H. G., Tarakeshwar, N. (2000). Negative religious coping predicts mortality among the medically ill. In: Annual Meeting of the American Psychological Association, 2000. Washington, DC: American Psychological Association.

Pargament, K. I., Tarakeshwar, N., Ellison, C. G., & Wulff, K. M. (2001). Religious coping among the religious: The relationships between religious coping and well-being in a national sample of Presbyterian clergy, elders, and members. *Journal for the scientific study of religion*, *40*(3), 497-513.

Powell, L. H., Shahabi, L., & Thoresen, C. E. (2003). Religion and spirituality: Linkages to physical health. *American psychologist*, *58*(1), 36.

Shahabi, L., Powell, L. H., Musick, M. A., Pargament, K. I., Thoresen, C. E., Williams, D., Underwood, L., Ory, M. A. (2002). Correlates of self-perceptions of spirituality in American adults. *Annals of Behavioral Medicine*, *24*(1), 59-68.

Shafranske, E. P. (1996). Religious beliefs, affiliations, and practices of clinical psychologists.

Shanafelt, T. D., Boone, S., Tan, L., Dyrbye, L. N., Sotile, W., Satele, D., ... & Oreskovich, M. R. (2012). Burnout and satisfaction with work-life balance among US physicians relative to the general US population. *ArcHIVes of internal medicine*, *172*(18), 1377-1385.

Tai-Seale, M., McGuire, T. G., & Zhang, W. (2007). Time allocation in primary care office visits. *Health services research*, *42*(5), 1871-1894.

Ward, L. C. (1995). Religion and Science Are Mutually Exclusive, *American Psychologist*, 50(7), 542-543.

Weaver, A. J., Samford, J. A., Larson, D. B., Lucas, L. A., Koenig, H. G., & Patrick, V. (1998). A systematic review of research on religion in four major psychiatric journals: 1991-1995. *The Journal of nervous and mental disease*, *186*(3), 187-189.

Chapter 3

RELIGION IN MODERN SOCIETY

Religious involvement remains a cornerstone of American society and deeply influences all aspects of moral and social life. In a 2010 Gallup poll, when asked the question, "Is religion an important part of your daily life?" 65% of Americans answered positively (Crabtree 2010). This is greater than similar western countries. In the United Kingdom, only 27% felt that religion was important for their daily life: in France, 30%, and Germany 40% (Crabtree, 2010). While Americans are more religious than most European countries, we are not quite as devoted to religious services as people who live in the developing world. 99% of the citizens of Bangladesh, Niger, Yemen, Indonesia, Malawi, and Sri Lanka agree that religion is an important part of daily life (Crabtree, 2010). Interestingly, in North America, we are much more religious than Canada where 42% agreed that religion was important to their daily lives, but not as much as our neighbors in Mexico (73%) (Crabtree, 2010). There is much speculation about this. Does wealth breed complacency? Does the rushed culture of a developed country crowd out the importance of religion?

And yet, religion remains an important aspect of American life. In another Gallup poll, 86% of the population believes in God and 85% believe in heaven. 54% are a member of a religious organization (Gallup, 2014). About the Bible, in 2014, 28% believe that the Bible was the "actual word" of God, and 47% believe the Bible is the "inspired word" of God. Also, American generally believe that religion is good for society. 75% believe that it would be positive for our country if we were more religious (Gallup, 2016). While there is generally belief and positive sentiment, in 2014, only 33% of the population attended religious services at least once a week, and 8% almost every week

(Newport, 2014). There is wide variety in religiosity in the country. In Mississippi, 63% consider themselves "very religious" while only 20% do in New Hampshire (Newport, 2016).

The religious landscape of America is complex and rapidly shifting. 50% of the population considers itself protestant while 24% are Catholic. In 1956, the peak that Gallup records, 71% considered themselves protestant and 25% were Catholic. Since then, the religious landscape of America has changed a great deal. Today, the fastest growing religious group is the "nones" – those who do not claim any religious affiliation. In 1956, the "nones" accounted for 1% of the population, and in 2015 account for 17%. For those under 30 years of age, those without a religious affiliation are 30% (Gallup, 2015).

Further, the evangelical movement seems to be in flux with some conflicting data. In 1998, 47% of Americans considered themselves to be "born again." In 2015, although not insignificant, only 38% were "born again." (Gallup, 2015) At the same time, "mega-churches" – those with more than 2,000 members – seem to be increasing their numbers. There are approximately 1,200 such churches. From 2009 to 2014, their attendance increased a median of 26% (Thuma, 2015).

The other recent revelation is that the "mainline churches" were never as "mainline" as previously believed. The mainline churches are characterized as those protestant denominations with long-standing presence in American culture. These are the religions of America's original European settlers: the English Episcopalians, Puritans, and Methodists, the Dutch Reformed, the German Lutherans, the Scottish Presbyterians. For the past 30 years, their membership has been in steady decline. In the early 1950's, membership peaked at approximately 40 million. By 2014, membership declined to approximately 15 million – a staggering 63%. Further, recent research shows that these mainline denominations counted only 16% of the American population in 1925 and decreased to 8.7% in 2000 (Campbell, 2014). These denominations may not have enjoyed a perceived cultural hegemony and outsized influence as initially believed; the religious landscape has been quite diverse for many generations.

In addition to religious diversity, there is diversity in *intensity* of belief and practice. While 69% of Americans self-reported that religion was important to their lives, on average 40% of them were in church the previous Sunday. This percentage varies widely by state. In Utah, the percentage is 41%, in Vermont, 17%. Given that 18-23% of the American population identifies no religious preference, this leaves a great percentage of the population somewhere in the middle.

This is bewildering for the healthcare provider who seeks to be culturally attuned to the needs of our patients. It is not enough to check a box recording religious preference. Interestingly, the religious commitment of physicians shows a higher percentage of atheists and agnostics than mainstream society. A study among Vermont family practitioners puts the prevalence of agnosticism or atheism at 36% (Maugans & Wadland, 1991). Among psychologists the prevalence is 28%, and among psychiatrists 21% (Bergin & Jensen, 1990).

What does this mean for the healthcare provider? In means, simply stated, that we should ask. Religion is as important as all the other important pieces of a patient's history: our family history, our support systems, our sexual practices, our cigarettes, our alcohol use. We should ask because the religious life of our patients is important to them. Their religion influences their decision-making about medication compliance and end-of-life care, family planning, and their approach to technology. Religion is important to our patients. We should ask.

REFERENCES

Bergin, A. E., & Jensen, J. P. (1990). Religiosity of psychotherapists: A national survey. *Psychotherapy: Theory, Research, Practice, Training*, *27*(1), 3.

Campbell, T., A. (2014). Glory days? The myth of the mainline. The Christian Century, 131(14), 11-13.

Crabtree, S. (2010). Religiosity Highest in World's Poorest Nations, retrieved February 10th, 2016 from http://www.gallup.com/poll/142727/religiosity-highest-world-poorest-nations.aspx.

Gallup. (2014, December 12). Seven in 10 Americans are very or moderately religious, Retrieved February 10th, 2016 from http://www.gallup.com/poll/159050/seven-americans-moderately-religious.aspx?utm_source=religion &utm_medium=search&utm_ campaign=tiles.

Gallup. (2015). Religion. Retrieved February 10th, 2016 from http://www.gallup.com/poll/1690/religion.aspx,

Maugans, T. A., & Wadland, W. C. (1991). Religion and family medicine: a survey of physicians and patients. *Journal of Family Practice*, *32*(2), 210-214.

Newport, F. (2014). Three Quarters of America Identify as Christian, retrieved February 1st, 2016, from http://www.gallup.com/poll/180347/three-quarters-americans-identify-christian.aspx?g_source=RELIGION_AND_SOCIAL_TRENDS&g_medium = topic&g_campaign = tiles.

Newport, F. (2016). New Hampshire Now Least Religious State, retrieved February 1st, 2016, from http://www.gallup.com/poll/189038/new-hampshire-least-religious-state.aspx?g_source=RELIGION&g_medium= topic&g_campaign = tiles.

Thuma, S., Bird, W. (2015). Recent Shifts in America's Largest Protestant Churchs: Megachurches 2015 Report, Leadership Network and Hartford Institute.

Chapter 4

Religion and Health Outcomes

With so many participating in religious organizations and so many with devote belief, the question is, "Does it make a difference to health?" What are the benefits, if any, of regular worship attendance, meditation, or prayerful practices? Is there any harm? While there are ample studies that address this, most of the data are correlation-type, observational studies. There remain very few intervention studies given the complex nature of studying this field.

Religion and Longevity

An important project that analyzed data from the National Health Interview Study, that included 22,080 subjects, discovered that mortality decreased with increased religious attendance. People who had never attended church were 19 times as likely to die as those who attended more than once a week over an 8-year period. (Hummer, 1999) Life expectancy is also prolonged among those who attend services more than once a week. Controlling for other factors, for people 20 years old, they can expect to live an average of 7 more years if they attend services more than once a week. This association was even stronger among African Americans who gained 13.7 years of life (Hummer et al., 1999). People who never attended religious services had a 1.87-fold increased risk of death when compared to people who attend services once per week (Hummer et al., 1999). Hummer speculates that the mechanism is through increased social ties and positive health behaviors.

A meta-analysis of 126,000 people, that incorporated 42 studies, and adjusted for other confounding variables, found that the odds of being alive at follow-up increased by 26% (McCullough et al., 2000). A classic study by Comstock et al., (1972) showed that people who did not attend religious services were 4 times as likely to commit suicide. Another study that demonstrated improved mortality was a 5 year follow up study among 2,025 residents of Marin Country who were 55 years of age and older. After 5 years, those with the lowest mortality were weekly church participants. Those with the highest mortality were the non-participants. An important feature of this study was that it controlled for other social activities that may confer similar social support, such as the Rotary Club, hospital auxiliaries, and other social clubs (Oman & Reed, 1998).

In an interesting study among nearly 600 severely ill hospitalized patients more than 55 years old, spiritual coping via a connection with God and receiving religious support was associated with less depression, better quality of life and greater compliance with care (Koenig 1998). This last point is particularly important: religiosity was associated with increased compliance with care. In an era where religion and science seem at odds, our patient's spiritual lives may actually be a tool towards accepting their medical care.

Since many of the cohort studies and surveys correlate religiosity with various psychological and physical factors, it can be difficult to imply causation. Randomized, or at least, longitudinal studies, are needed. There has been a growing literature that has evaluated this. Oman and colleagues (1995) prospectively evaluated 6 month mortality among patients undergoing open heart surgery. He found that mortality was significantly higher among those who did not receive strength and comfort from their religious faith when compared with more religious patients. In a prospective study among 400 elderly patients, regular religious attendance was associated with lower mortality at 2-year follow up. (Zuckerman, 1984) Strawbridge found that religious attendance reduced 28-year mortality risk among community dwelling residents in Alameda County, California. Idler and Kasl (1992) found that elderly residents in New Haven, CT may delay their death until after the conclusion of major religious holidays.

Religious Involvement, Blood Pressure and Lipids

Other studies assess how religious involvement has other systemic effects in the body's chemistry. Koenig et al., (1998) showed that religious involvement lowered blood pressure. In a sample of 3,963 individuals, people who attended religious services once a week had a small, but statistically significant lower systolic and diastolic blood pressures (1-4mm Hg). Blood pressure differences were markedly lower among African American and elderly attendees. Lower blood pressure was also observed among those who prayed or studied the Bible regularly. They also found a dose effect. Among participants who attended religious services and prayed or studied the Bible frequently were 40% less likely to have diastolic hypertension (Koenig et al., 1998).

Other studies have shown similar findings. In an ingenious study, Steffen et al. (2001) studied 24 ambulatory blood pressure readings among 155 men and women. Among African Americans, those who employed greater religious coping had lower blood pressure readings (Steffen et al., 2001). Another study among 407 men showed that religious importance, independent of church attendance, was associated with lower blood pressure. There seemed to be a dose effect: those with the lowest blood pressure attended church regularly and placed a high importance on religion. These effects remained significant even after controlling for weight-height ratio, smoking, and socioeconomic status (Larson et al., 1989). In a case control study, Timio et al., (1997) studied a cohort of nuns and a matched control of lay women in the same region of Umbria, Italy over a period of 30 years. They found that the nuns' blood pressure remained stable throughout while the lay women had an expected age-related elevation of blood pressure, resulting in a statistically significant difference of 30/15 ($p < .001$) (Timio et al., 1997).

Several studies have shown how religious participation improved lipid profiles. Friedlander et al., (1985) studied a population of Jewish residents in Jerusalem. Those who self-identified as being more religious had lower lipid levels in comparison to those who self-identified as being secular. Friedlander speculates that this may have been due to dietary and other health influences: secular Jews consumed more fat, and were more likely to smoke than religious subjects (Friedlander, 1985). Friedlander (Friedlander, Kark, & Stein, 1987) also studied 673 Jewish teenagers of Jerusalem. He compared orthodox Jews, traditional Jews, and nonobservant Jews. When controlling for gender, social class, body mass index, and season, orthodox Jews had lower cholesterol, triglycerides, and low-density lipoprotein levels than secular children (Friedlander, Kark, & Stein, 1987). These studies are particularly provocative since the study population is largely uniform: all were Jewish living in Jerusalem. Yet, their personal practices were different. While some of the difference may be ascribed to dietary influence, these effects cannot be accounted for diet alone.

Meditation, Mindfulness and Health Outcomes

While there are relatively few studies that measure such health indices among based on religiosity, there are a wealth of studies that study the influence of mindfulness and meditation. Perhaps the earliest study that spawned this research was by Herbert Benson et al., (1974) who studied 14 subjects with hypertension. During a control period, he showed no change in blood pressure, which averaged 145.6/91.9. He then taught the subjects transcendental meditation. During the 20 week experimental period where subjects regularly practiced transcendental meditation, systolic blood pressure dropped to 135 ($p < .01$) and diastolic blood pressure dropped to 87 ($p < .05$) (Benson et al., 1974). Of note, this paper was published in *The Lancet*, one of the most prestigious journals in the world. This paper heralded wide-spread interest in this field of meditation and its effects on health. Several studies soon followed.

Other meditation and relaxation exercises have been shown to lower cholesterol and blood pressure. Patel et al., (1985) performed a randomized controlled trial among older adults with hypertension and hypercholesterolemia. The control arm was given a leaflet about healthy habits. The intervention arm was taught meditation and breathing exercises one hour a week for 8 weeks. At the end of the 8 weeks, there was a statistically significant drop in their lipids and blood pressure compared to the control group. Interestingly, this effect persisted at a four years of follow up. Patients in the control arm had greater incidence of angina and fatal myocardial infarction (Patel et al., 1985). Another randomized trial evaluated those patients with angiographically proven coronary artery disease (Manchanda et al., 2000). The control group ($n = 21$) was managed by conventional methods – the step 1 American Heart Association Diet and risk factor control. The intervention group ($n = 21$) was taught a "user friendly" program of yoga, relaxation techniques, and moderate exercise. Angiography repeated at one year showed more lesions had regressed (20% vs 2%, $p = .01$, $p < .0001$) and less lesions progressed (5% vs 37%, $p < .0001$) in the yoga group. Similarly, revascularization procedures were less frequently required in the yoga group (1 vs 8, relative risk 5.45, $p = .01$) (Machanda et al., 2000).

NEGATIVE STUDIES IN THE DISCIPLINE OF SPIRITUALITY AND HEALTH

While there is strong evidence about the healthful effects of religiosity and spirituality for our patients, it is important to have a balanced view. There are significant issues with religion that directly impact health. Religion is a charged subject politically, and even among close friends, religion can be a dicey topic in conversation. As such, it is a challenge for researchers not to have a bias. Many look for positive associations. Some seek negative associations. Some researchers suggest that certain forms of religiosity can have a detrimental effect on health. Religion can be alienating, can justify hatred, aggression, and prejudice, and can be a source of guilt, negative interpersonal experiences, and congregational criticism (Williams & Sternthal, 2007).

There is a social dynamic that, for the most part, is supportive and helpful. However, some religious-based social relationships can be a source of stress (Ano & Vasconcelles, 2005). "Are you measuring up? Are you giving enough? Why did you miss the church potluck?" Failure to meet community norms can lead to feelings of guilt and unworthiness. Parents' reliance on faith healing and interventional prayer has led to the death and significant morbidity of some children (Asser & Swan, 1998).

Religion is not always associated with lower depression. An important paper by Smith et al., (2003), who is generally supportive of religion, showed that an extrinsic religious orientation (i.e., Regular worship attendance) in combination with a negative religious coping attitude (i.e., The belief that "God is punishing me") is associated with elevated symptoms of depression (Smith, McCullough, & Poll, 2003). Congregational criticism and negative interpersonal experiences at church have been associated with increased depression among adolescents (Cotton et al., 2006).

A longitudinal study that followed medically ill patients for 2 years found that religious doubts and struggle were associated with greater mortality (Pargament et al., 2001). Since food is so often an important social dimension to religious life, several studies have explored the possibility of obesity – with it's concomitant health impact - among religious participants. One study showed that body-mass-index varied by religious denomination and that increased religious attendance was associated with greater weight (Ferraro, 1998). However, a follow up study found that such an association could be explained by controlling for socio-demographic and health variables. (Kim, 2007).

A study by Van Wagoner et al., (2014) evaluated religious men who contracted HIV infection by having intercourse with other men. He showed that religious men with HIV infection presented later in their illness with poorer immune status. The authors speculate that this was due, in part, to their church's unfavorable view of homosexuality (Van Wagoner et al., 2014). Also, Wanyama et al., (2007) evaluated HIV patients who had poor virologic control. 1.2% of those patients stopped their medications due to belief in "spiritual healing" – God had cured them of their HIV. And yet, they showed evidence of advancing illness. While this represented only a small percentage of treatment failures, it nonetheless remains an important consideration for the provider.

Religious Attendance and Life Satisfaction

Church attendance has been positively associated with improved life satisfaction than those who self-identify as being atheists (Donovan & Halpern, 2002; Ellison & Levin, 1998). Religiously active people also tend to be happier, live longer, and have lower suicide rates (Helliwell & Putnam, 2005; McIntosh & Spilka, 1990). While some of the variation may be due to religious precepts against drinking and cigarette smoking, the effect on behavior is incomplete (McCullough et al., 2000).

But what is it about religion that closely ties it to improved well-being? Is not feeling a connection to God, feeling that God answers prayers, and feeling connected to others simply another marker for subjective well-being and life satisfaction? Are they measuring the same thing? Yes and no. While there is some degree of overlap, religiosity is not the same as subjective well-being. Some models are proposed to account for this positive effect of religion. Ardelt (2003) suggests that it is purpose in life, and not intrinsic or extrinsic religiosity, that is protective to preserves well-being. Ellison and Levin (1998) suggest that religion provides an interpretive framework that makes sense of life experience. Helliwell and Putnam (2005) have suggested that religious involvement generates community bonds and social capital that fosters well-being.

THE PRACTICE OF FAITH AND DISEASE

Religion is multi-dimensional. While there are neuro-chemical associations with religious involvement, there are also social norms around diet, sexuality, and the prohibition against alcohol and drugs that impact our patient's health. Interesting studies among the Seventh-day Adventist and Mormon communities has shown several positive effects. Both and Mormons and Adventists prohibit alcohol and tobacco; and the Adventists encourage vegetarianism. Both faith communities have lower rates of hypertension, cardiovascular disease, and cancer (Rouse, Armstrong, & Beilin, 1982). The Seventh Day Adventists also have lower rates of obesity (Armstrong, Van Merwyk, & Coates, 1977; Fraser, 1999).

Several healthy behaviors, that have no specific religious precepts, appear more commonly among those who practice their religion. For example, a large study among high school seniors found that those who were more religious were more likely to wear seatbelts, eat breakfast, eat green vegetables and fruit, get regular exercise, and sleep at least 7 hours a night (Wallace & Forman, 1998). Religious participation may offer a perspective and moderating influence on healthy behaviors. Religious participation may also be a marker for compliance in other healthy behaviors: religious people comply with their religious teachings and so are more compliant in other social norms. Participation in religious communities also has been shown to provide support and a sense of connectedness, which led to positive changes in health behaviors over time (Strawbridge et al., 2001).

CONCLUSION

Religious involvement and spiritual attitudes are complex constructs. There is a deep personal dimension. What does a patient believe? What is their worldview? There is also a practice to religion and spirituality. Does a patient pray? Meditate? Does a patient's religious belief manifest itself in certain diet and other health-related practices? And there is a social dimension. How does a patient interact with one's religious community? There are normative affects that are largely positive. People feel affirmed in their religious communities. There is also a population bias; those who are not supported by their religious communities leave to seek other community. The gay male, for example, might feel ostracized from a socially conservative church. And yet, religion and spirituality matters. It makes a difference to people's lives. It can be helpful to discern *why* religion and spirituality make a difference. Is it belief? Prayerful practice? Community? But, it is perhaps more important that it *does* make a difference. These studies – and there are many more – make a difference to our patients' longevity and overall health. If there were a pill that would reduce heart disease, without side effects, we would certainly prescribe it. And yet, this is precisely the case with religious and spiritual involvement: it makes a difference. Exploring this resource is important to our work as healthcare providers.

REFERENCES

Ano, G. G., & Vasconcelles, E. B. (2005). Religious coping and psychological adjustment to stress: A meta-analysis. *Journal of clinical psychology, 61*(4), 461-480.

Ardelt, M. (2003). Effects of religion and purpose in life on elders' subjective well-being and attitudes towards death. *Journal of Religious Gerontology,* 14(4), 55–77.

Armstrong, B., Van Merwyk, A. J., & Coates, H. (1977). Blood pressure in Seventh-day Adventist vegetarians. *American Journal of Epidemiology, 105*(5), 444-449.

Asser, S. M., & Swan, R. (1998). Child fatalities from religion-motivated medical neglect. *Pediatrics, 101*(4), 625-629.

Benson, H., Marzetta, B., Rosner, B., & Klemchuk, H. (1974). Decreased blood-pressure in pharmacologically treated hypertensive patients who regularly elicited the relaxation response. *The Lancet, 303*(7852), 289-291.

Comstock, G. W., & Partridge, K. B. (1972). Church attendance and health. Journal of chronic diseases, *25*(12), 665-672.

Cotton, S., Zebracki, K., Rosenthal, S. L., Tsevat, J., Drotar, D., (2006). Religion/spirituality and adolescent health outcomes: a review, *Journal of Adolescent Health.* 38, 472-480

Donovan, N., & Halpern, D. (2002). Life satisfaction: The state of knowledge and implications for government, analytical paper. London: Strategy Unit.

Ellison, C. G., & Levin, J. S. (1998). The religion–health connection: Evidence, theory, and future directions. *Health Education and Behavior,* 25(6), 700–720.

Ferraro, K. F. (1998). Firm believers? Religion, body weight, and well-being. *Review of Religious Research*, 224-244.

Fraser, G. E. (1999). Diet as primordial prevention in Seventh-Day Adventists. *Preventive medicine*, *29*(6), S18-S23.

Friedlander, Y., Kark, J. D., Kaufmann, N. A., & Stein, Y. (1985). Coronary heart disease risk factors among religious groupings in a Jewish population sample in Jerusalem. *American Journal of Clinical Nutrition, 42,* 511–521.

Friedlander, Y., Kark, J. D., & Stein, Y. (1987). Religious observance and plasma lipids and lipoproteins among 17-year-old Jewish residents of Jerusalem. *Preventive Medicine, 16,* 70–79.

Helliwell, J. F., & Putnam, R. D. (2005). The social context of well-being. In F. A. Huppert, N. Baylis, & B. Kevern (Eds.), The science of well-being (pp. 435–460). Oxford: Oxford University Press.

Hummer, R. A., Rogers, R. G., Nam, C. B., Ellison, CB. (1999). Religious involvement and US adult mortality, *Demography*, 36(2):273-85.

Kim, K. H. C. (2007). Religion, weight perception, and weight control behavior. *Eating Behaviors*, *8*(1), 121-131.

Koenig, H. G., George, L. K., Hays, J. C., Larson, D. B., Cohen, H. J., & Blazer, D. G. (1998). The relationship between religious activities and blood pressure in older adults. *The International Journal of Psychiatry in Medicine*, *28*(2), 189-213.

Larson, D. B., Koenig, H. G., Kaplan, B. H., Greenberg, R. S., Logue, E.,& Tyroler, H. A. (1989). The impact of religion on men's blood pressure. *Journal of Religion and Health, 28,* 265–278.

McCullough, M. E., Hoyt, W. T., Larson, D. B., Koenig, H. G., & Thoresen, C. (2000). Religious involvement and mortality: a meta-analytic review. *Health psychology*, *19*(3), 211.

Manchanda, S. C., Narang, R., Reddy, K. S., Sachdeva, U., Prabhakaran, D., Dharmanand, S., ... & Bijlani, R. (2000). Retardation of coronary atherosclerosis with yoga lifestyle intervention. *The Journal of the Association of Physicians of India*, *48*(7), 687-694.

McIntosh, D. N., & Spilka, B. B. (1990). Religion and physical health: The role of personal faith and control beliefs. In M. L. Lynn, & D. O. Moberg (Eds.), Research on the social scientific study of religion (Vol. 2, pp. 167–194). Greenwich: JAI Press.

Oman, D., & Reed, D. (1998). Religion and mortality among the community-dwelling elderly. *American Journal of Public Health*, *88*(10), 1469-1475.

Patel, C., Marmot, M. G., Terry, D. J., Carruthers, M., Hunt, B., & Patel, M. (1985). Trial of relaxation in reducing coronary risk: Four year follow up. *British Medical Journal, 290,* 1103–1106.

Pargament, K. I., Koenig, H. G., Tarakeshwar, N., & Hahn, J. (2001). Religious struggle as a predictor of mortality among medically ill elderly patients: A 2-year longitudinal study. *ArcHIVes of internal Medicine*, *161*(15), 1881-1885.

Rouse, I. L., Armstrong, B. K., & Beilin, L. J. (1982). Vegetarian diet, lifestyle and blood pressure in two religious populations. *Clinical and Experimental Pharmacology and Physiology*, *9*(3), 327-330.

Smith, T. B., McCullough, M. E., & Poll, J. (2003). Religiousness and depression: evidence for a main effect and the moderating influence of stressful life events. *Psychological bulletin*, *129*(4), 614.

Steffen, P. R., Hinderliter, A. L., Blumenthal, J. A., & Sherwood, A. (2001). Religious coping, ethnicity, and ambulatory blood pressure. *Psychosomatic Medicine, 63,* 523–530.

Strawbridge, W. J., Shema, S. J., Cohen, R. D., & Kaplan, G. A. (2001). Religious attendance increases survival by improving and maintaining good health behaviors, mental health, and social relationships. *Annals of Behavioral Medicine*, *23*(1), 68-74.

Timio, M., Lippi, G., Venanzi, S., Gentili, S., Quintaliani, G., Verdura, C., ... & Timio, F. (1997). Blood pressure trend and cardiovascular events in nuns in a secluded order: a 30-year follow-up study. *Blood Pressure*, *6*(2), 81-87.

Van Wagoner, N., Mugavero, M., Westfall, A., Hollimon, J., Slater, L. Z., Burkholder, G., Raper, J., & Hook, E. W. (2014). Church attendance in men who have sex with men diagnosed with HIV is associated with later presentation for HIV care. *Clinical Infectious Diseases*, *58*(2), 295-299.

Wallace, J. M., & Forman, T. A. (1998). Religion's role in promoting health and reducing risk among American youth. *Health Education & Behavior*, *25*(6), 721-741.

Wanyama, J., Castelnuovo, B., Wandera, B., Mwebaze, P., Kambugu, A., Bangsberg, D. R., & Kamya, M. R. (2007). Belief in divine healing can be a barrier to antiretroviral therapy adherence in Uganda. *Aids*, *21*(11), 1486-1487.

Williams, D. R., & Sternthal, M. J. (2007). Spirituality, religion and health: Evidence and research directions. *Medical Journal of Australia*, 186(10), 47–50.

Chapter 5

The Biology of Religion and Spirituality

Much of the data on religion and health outcomes are associations only. Religious people tend to live longer, suffer less depression, and recover more quickly from surgeries. An important aspect of this observed outcome is the influence that religion and spirituality has on our biological processes. As sociological studies became more prevalent, researchers began exploring the biochemical effects of religiosity. There are several provocative studies that would compel even the most ardent skeptic to consider religious involvement as a means to health. The study of the biological mechanisms of religiosity can be understood to affect the brain, as well as neurotransmitters, the endocrine system, and the immune response, where the most important stress hormones are dopamine, epinephrine, and norepinephrine. In general, any practice that fosters lower levels of stress hormones and inflammatory cytokines will have healthful effects.

The Brain

Prayer and meditation have been shown through functional MRI imaging to mediate important brain structures that are associated with wellness, including the frontal lobe, limbic system, hypothalamus, and amygdala (McNamara, Andresen, & Gellard, 2003). Functional magnetic resonance imagining (fMRI) demonstrates that patients who meditate have increased activity in the left hemisphere, which has been associated with a positive mood, improved immune response as measured by antibody titers and natural killer cell activity (Kang et al., 1991, Davidson et al., 2003).

Religious activity has been shown to activate the prefrontal cortex – a region of the brain that is associated with executive functions, meaning, optimism, and construction. Part of this effect is mediated through the increased activity of dopamine at the level of the prefrontal cortex - a richly enervated area which is associated with positive rewards. Interestingly, this is the same pathway that addicting drugs activate to produce their rewarding effects (McNamara 2002). Activation of the prefrontal cortex is also important for the development of appropriate behaviors and attitudes – such as impulse control, empathy, and self-responsibility.

A very provocative study evaluated the neuroplasticity of 20 subjects who incorporated regular meditation into their daily work and family life. The study found that those areas of the brain associated with attention and sensory processing - like the pre-frontal cortex – were thicker in comparison to matched controls. This effect was most pronounced in older participants, suggesting that meditation might offset age-related cortical thinning (Lazar et al., 2005). This study suggests that meditation can actually cause structural changes to the brain. Another meditation study by Jevning et al., (1996) showed that meditation techniques increased cerebral blood flow and decreased cerebrovascular resistance.

Stress Hormones and the Immune Response

In other functional MRI studies, religious behavior and attitudes have been shown to activate the prefrontal cortex and to increase activity in the hippocampus and amygdale. The locus coeruleus also delivers less noradrenaline to the hypothalamic paraventricular nucleus (PVN) and decreases the production of corticotrophin releasing hormone (CRH) and cortisol. The urine and plasma studies show decreased cortisol level during meditation. Meditation increases parasympathetic activity which leads to a decrease in heart rate and respiratory rate and the subjective sensation of relaxation and then later a deeper sense of quiescence (Newberg & Iversen, 2003). Meditation has also been shown to increase serotonin, dopamine, and endorphins, reduce cortisone and cortisone releasing hormone (Newberg and Iverson 2003).

A study by King et al., (2002) used the National Health and Nutrition Examination Survey III (1988-1994) to evaluate 556 people with diabetes and the relationship between c-reactive protein and religious participation. C-reactive protein is an inflammatory marker that portends worse cardiovascular morbidity. King et al., (2002) found that, among people with diabetes, those who did not attend religious services were more likely to have an elevated C-reactive protein (Odds Ratio 2.17 (95% CI 1.1504.09).

A study by Koenig et al., (1997) examined the relationship between religious attendance among older adults and IL-6, a marker of inflammation. When controlling for socio-demographic variables, regular attendance was associated with lower IL-6 levels, suggesting a healthier overall immune system (Koenig et al., 1997).

Meditation, prayer, religious commitment cause healthful, positive changes within the brain and the body's chemsitry. Karl Marx said, "Religion is the opium of the people."[2] In one sense, he is right: religious involvement does affect the same parts of the brain that opium and other substances impact with increased "feel good" hormones and a lower stress response . However, many studies show deleterious effects on the brain with abuse of opium and alcohol (Di Sclafani et al., 2002). These studies pertaining to religion and spirituality demonstrate the same improvement in mood without the deleterious effects of addiction, destruction of brain pathways, and risks to health.

Heightened sympathetic activation has been shown to cause poor cardiac outcomes due to increased platelet aggregation, increased coagulation, and recurrent thrombus formation (Frasure-Smith, Lesperance, & Talajic, 1995). Increased catecholamines can increase heart rate variability, which leads to cardiac dysrhythmias. Further, catecholamines lead to increased vasoconstriction, which accelerates arteriosclerosis and promotes endothelial dysfunction. This leads to decreased coronary blood flow.

Meditation also decreases norepinephrine and increases levels of glutamate and gamma-aminobutyric acid (GABA), which are important neurotransmitters that mediate relaxation (Walton et al., 1995). Interestingly, if glutamate levels are too high, the brain slows down production. This allows for an accumulation of a glutamate precursor – N-acetylated-a-linked-acidic dipeptidase (NAAG). This substance is a hallucinogenic, causing similar dissociative sensations as ketamine and phencyclidine. This is the substance believed to be responsible for out-of-body and mystical experiences (Thomas

[2] The full quote is, "Religion is the sigh of the oppressed creature, the heart of a heartless world, and the soul of soulless conditions. It is the opium of the people." Marx, K, A Contribution to the Critique of Hegel's Philosophy of Right (1844).

et al., 2000). Some researches implicate the serotonin system as a biological basis for spiritual experiences (Borg et al., 2003).

Several studies have investigated brain function and spirituality. One important study evaluated the brain function of 12 healthy volunteers: six were religious, six non-religious. Imaging studies reveal that religious experience involves a neural-circuit that involves a complex interplay between the higher structures of the brain – the frontal and prefrontal cortex – and the more rudimentary structures such as the limbic system and amygdale (Azari, 2001).

Some studies have shown that the temporal-limbic system is a substrate of religious-numinous experience (Pietrini, 2003). In functional MRI studies, the right temporal lobe is activated during mystical states, while the left temporal lobe is activated during religious delusions (Pietrini, 2003; Fenwick, 2001).

Religious experiences have often been characterized as "temporal lobe dysfunction," since the temporal lobe epilepsy is often the locus of hallucinations, déjà vu experiences, and spatial dysphoria (Saver & Rabin, 1997). The temporal lobe seems also to connect deeper meaning to ordinary experiences. However, a rebuttal to this "temporal lobe" dysfunction points out that no literature has demonstrated a reduction in religious sentiment among patients who have had their temporal lobes damaged or removed.

These studies are important for several reasons. They demonstrate compelling evidence that religious involvement in all its forms – from personal devotional practices meditation to corporate worship – have healthful effects on our body's biochemistry. Several of these studies are generalized to practices that are not associated with a specific religious tradition. Yoga and meditation, for example, have distinct religious origins, but now have joined a secular mainstream. And yet, if one were to have a "dose" of healthful practices, why not religion?

These studies are compelling to a patient who is pondering what next to try in regaining their health, treating their depression, or improving their mind. It seems our brain is, quite literally, wired for religion. In my opinion, studies that address brain function and neuro-chemistry merely describe at the molecular level what we know to be true at the physiologic level. Religiosity, in general, is good for health.

REFERENCES

Azari, N. P., Nickel, J., Wunderlich, G., Niedeggen, M., Hefter, H., Tellmann, L., ... & Seitz, R. J. (2001). Neural correlates of religious experience. *European Journal of Neuroscience*, *13*(8), 1649-1652.

Borg, J., Bengt, A., Soderstrom, H., Farde, L. (2003). The serotonin system and spiritual experiences. American Journal of Psychiatry 160, 1965–9.

Davidson, R. J., Kabat-Zinn, J., Schumacher, J., Rosenkranz, M., Muller, D., Santorelli, S. F., ... & Sheridan, J. F. (2003). Alterations in brain and immune function produced by mindfulness meditation. *Psychosomatic medicine*, *65*(4), 564-570.

Di Sclafani, V., Tolou-Shams, M., Price, L. J., & Fein, G. (2002). Neuropsychological performance of individuals dependent on crack–cocaine, or crack–cocaine and alcohol, at 6 weeks and 6 months of abstinence. *Drug and alcohol dependence*, *66*(2), 161-171.

Fenwick, P. (2001). The neurophysiology of religious experience. In: Clarke I, ed. psychosis and spirituality: exploring the new frontier. (pp. 15-26) London: Whurr Publishers Ltd.

Frasure-Smith, N., Lesperance, F., & Talajic, M. (1995). The impact of negative emotions on prognosis following myocardial infarction: is it more than depression?. *Health Psychology*, *14*(5), 388.

Jevning, R., Anand, R., Biedebach, M., & Fernando, G. (1996). Effects on regional blood flow of transcendental meditation. *Physiology and Behavior, 59,* 399–402.

Kang, D. H., Davidson, R. J., Coe, C. L., Wheeler, R. E., Tomarken, A. J., & Ershler, W. B. (1991). Frontal brain asymmetry and immune function. *Behavioral Neuroscience*, 105, 860–869.

King, D. E., Mainous, A. G., & Pearson, W. S. (2002). C-reactive protein, diabetes, and attendance at religious services. *Diabetes Care*, *25*(7), 1172-1176.

Koenig, H. G., Cohen, H. J., George, L. K., Hays, J. C., Larson, D. B., & Blazer, D. G. (1997). Attendance at religious services, interleukin-6, and other biological parameters of immune function in older adults. *International Journal of Psychiatry in Medicine, 27,* 233–250.

Lazar S. W., Kerr C. E., Wasserman R. H., Gray J. R., Greve D. N., Treadway M. T., McGarvey M., Quinn B. T., Dusek J. A., Benson H., Rauch S. L., Moore C. I., Fischl B., (2005). Meditation experience is associated with increased cortical thickness, *Neuroreport*, 16 (17), 1893-1897.

McNamara, P. (2002). The motivational origins of religious practices. Zygon, 37, 143–160.

McNamara, P., Andresen, J., & Gellard, J. (2003). Relation of religiosity and scores on fluency tests to subjective reports of health in older individuals. *The International Journal for the Psychology of Religion*, 13, 259–271.

Newberg A. B., Iversen J., (2003). The neural basis of the complex mental task of meditation: neurotransmitter and neurochemical considerations, *Medical Hypotheses*, 61: 2, 282-291.

Pietrini, P. (2003). Toward a biochemistry of mind? *American Journal of Psychiatry* 160, 1907–8.

Saver, J. L., & Rabin, J. (1997). The neural substrates of religious experience. *The neuropsychiatry of limbic and subcortical disorders*, 195-207.

Thomas, A. G., Vornov, J. J., Olkowski, J. L., Merion, A. T., & Slusher, B. S. (2000). N-acetylated α-linked acidic dipeptidase converts N-acetylaspartylglutamate from a neuroprotectant to a neurotoxin. *Journal of Pharmacology and Experimental Therapeutics*, *295*(1), 16-22.

Walton, K. G., Pugh, N. D., Gelderloos, P., & Macrae, P. (1995). Stress reduction and preventing hypertension: Preliminary support for a psychoneuroendocrine mechanism. *Journal of Alternative and Complementary Medicine, 1,* 263–283.

Chapter 6

THE SPIRITUAL LIVES OF CHILDREN

Studying the spiritual lives of children presents several challenges. What is the difference between fanciful thinking and "true" belief? Does it matter? Does a child's belief that God loves her and that she is safe from harm hopelessly naïve or a model of faith? If a child prays to God, is that an expression of faith? What if he talks to his "imaginary friend" or asks his stuffed animal for help? Is that pretend? It is difficult to tease apart these factors. In the same way, one wonders about the sophistication of "adult faith." If an adult believes our souls go to heaven when we die, is that fanciful thinking? Plato believed this to be true, and any number of saints and religious figures across many faith traditions believe this.

The other dimension to the study of religiosity in children is cultural. Children, for the most part, inherit the faith of their parents. There are cultural traditions, family values, and elements of togetherness that are unique to religion. The practice of religion, for a child more so than an adult, cannot be completely divested from intrinsic belief. Religiosity within a family, by itself, may be marker of other family values that may portend a positive outcome: family cohesion, traditional values, a sense of order and ritual in life.

But what of the personal beliefs of the child, especially an adolescent? If church is boring, oppressive, or too stuffy, does a child get any health benefit? Any benefit in terms of self-esteem or positive self image? And the contrary might be equally true: an oppressive church experience may convey negative self-images and result in lower self-esteem. What does the data say? For the most part, studies among the pediatric population focus on adolescents where faith and spirituality begin to have a distinct construct from child fantasy.

Further, most of the studies focus on the practice of religion and the attendance of religious services.

ADOLESCENCE, RELIGION AND HEALTH

Religion and spirituality are certainly important to adolescents. In several recent surveys, 95% believe in God. 85-95% affirm that religion is important in their life. 93% believe God loves them. 67% believe in life after death. 50% attend religious services at least monthly and participate in religious youth groups. Nearly half frequently pray alone (Smith et al., 2002; Gallup & Bezilla, 1992; Smith & Denton, 2005). In general, African-American and Hispanic youth are more religious than white youth. Female teenagers tend to be more religious than male teens. Younger adolescents tend to be more religious than older teens (Smith et al., 2002).

In an important systematic review, Rew and Wong (2006) found 43 studies from 1993-2003 that specifically addressed the issues of religiosity and spirituality among adolescent health attitudes and behaviors. Most of the studies (84%) showed a positive effect upon health attitudes and behaviors (Rew & Wong, 2006).

Adolescence is an age of comparable physical health. Among 15-19 year olds, mortality among from cancer is only 3.2 per 100,000 and ranks fourth behind accidents (31.3), homicide (10.8), and suicide (7.3). Thus, modulating risky behaviors is an important aspect to the care of the adolescent (Centers for Disease Control, 2006). And yet, 65% of adult mortality – namely stroke, heart disease, and cancer – are influenced by behaviors that begin in adolescence. Adolescence is an important time where patterns of wellness begin and have great impact in later years. For example, more than 15% of adolescents are obese. If a teenager is obese, there is an 80% likelihood that they will become an obese adult (Must & Strauss, 1999). Obesity, even in adolescents, has been shown to increase blood pressure, insulin, and lipid levels (Freedman et al., 1999).

More important is mental health, drug use, and teen pregnancy. 50% of high school students will have sexual intercourse, resulting in 25-33% of all sexually transmitted infections in the United States (Blum & Nelson-Mmari, 2004). 19% of teenage girls who have sexual intercourse will get pregnant. 30% of pregnancies are terminated, accounting for 20% of all abortions in the United States. The impact of teen pregnancy has enormous implications, including increased prevalence of poverty, school cessation, food stamp use, and other welfare programs (Dalby, Hayon, & Carlson, 2014).

Further, the use of alcohol and drugs among adolescents is quite high. Among 12-17 year olds, 15.9% drank alcohol, 9.5% used drugs, 6.7% smoked marijuana (Mulye et al., 2009). The prevalence of depression among adolescents is 2% with a cumulative incidence of 15-20% during the adolescent years. Depression is an important influence in alcohol use, suicide attempts, and promiscuity (Kessler, Avenevoli, & Merikangas, 2001). All of this is to say that, while adolescence is a time of general physical health, there are serious and widely prevalent risk-taking behaviors that can have a lasting-impact in their lives, their family's lives, and subsequent generations.

Religion, Mental Health and Behavior

Many studies evaluate attendance at religious services and self-reported "importance" of religion among the adolescent population and health outcomes. Perhaps one of the largest studies evaluated religious attendance and "importance" of religion among 69,340 students in high school. Wallace et al., (2003) found that increased attendance and "importance" of religion correlated with decreased alcohol and illicit drug use (Wallace et al., 2003).

Another study evaluated 451 patients with the Beck Depression Inventory. Adolescents who reported higher attendance at religious services and increased importance of religion had lower depression scores (Wright, Frost, & Wisecarver, 1993). Increased attendance and self-identified importance of religion also correlates with improved academic performance and college attendance (Regnerus, 2003). Other studies have shown that religious coping reduces nighttime fear among 8-12 year olds, improves outcomes in adolescents recovering from sexual abuse, hospitalized 8-10 year olds (Ollendick, Grills, & Alexander 2001).

Religion, then, can become an important modulating influence in the care of our adolescent patients. At a time with the influence of peer groups often outweigh the influence of parents and family, one's religious community can be an important resource. A religious community – in particular youth group, Sunday school or other age-oriented group activities – can offer a mid-way station between the shelter of family life and full autonomy. Religious life can offer mature relationships, supportive structure, and positive feedback that supports adolescent well-being.

Further, religious activities and religiosity in general seem to be protective against several risk taking health behaviors: including early sexual initiation, drug and alcohol use, and truancy. Higher levels of spirituality and religiosity seem to be protective against depression, poor body image, and other mental health problems (Wallace & Forman, 1998; Smith & Denton, 2005; Pearce, Little & Perez, 2003; Wright, Frost, and Wisecarver, 1993). In a longitudinal study among 7th-10th graders, Wills et al. (2003) found that religiosity was associated with lower use of alcohol, tobacco, and marijuana. Also, Lammers et al. (2000) found that greater religiosity was associated with lower levels of sexual behavior.

In the comprehensive cross-section study of adolescent health, which evaluated more than 12,000 teenagers from the National Longitudinal Study on Adolescent Health, showed that high levels of prayer and self-reported importance of religion correlated with lower frequency of cigarette use and later sexual debut (Resnick et al., 1997).

Spirituality and religiosity are shown to be protective in several health behaviors. Higher levels of spiritual connectedness and the use of spiritual coping were inversely related to voluntary sexual activity and substance use in several studies (Hodge, Cardenas, & Montoya, 2001; Holder et al., 2000; Ritt-Olson et al., 2004). The mechanism to this effect seems to be both the social connectedness of the spiritual community (i.e., a youth group) as well as an adolescent's intrinsic spiritual belief (Resnick, Harris, & Blum, 1993). This effect holds true across ethnic groups as well as ages (7th-12th grade) (Resnick, Harris, & Blum, 1993). Thus, it is not only the normative restrictions of the religious community, such as against drinking alcohol or engaging in premarital sexual activity. But, there are intrinsic values at play as well – such as one's relationship to the divine, regarding one's body as a temple, one's sense of intrinsic value – that also seems to reduce risk taking behavior.

Spirituality and religiosity has also been shown to be protective in the domain of mental health. In a study among 451 teenagers, Wright et al., (1993) found that those adolescents who had a greater value of religion in their lives and interactions with others had lower levels of depression ($p < .05$). Other studies among adolescents found that increased religious commitment and increased religious influence reduced drug and alcohol use, sexual activity, and also reduced the risk of suicide (Greening & Stoppelbein, 2002; Rew et al., 2001).

One interesting study explored the *quality* not the *quantity* of religious experience. In particular, negative or demanding interactions in one's religious congregation was associated with greater levels of depression. The converse was true as well. Those adolescents who experienced a positive interaction had lower prevalence of depression ($r = .15$, $p < .01$) (Pearce, Little, & Perez, 2003). Another study by Cotton et al., (2005) and colleagues echoed this finding. In a study among 134 suburban adolescents, the greater importance of religion was associated with greater prevalence of depression. (Cotton 2005) Instead of discounting these negative studies in the face of so many other positive ones, perhaps there are important lessons to learn. Could it be the content of the religious teachings? Could it be that depressed teenagers continue their depression despite the positive influence of the church community?

Interestingly, in two studies only the social experiences and the religious teachings were associated with lower depressive symptoms. More simplistic measurements of religiosity – such as church attendance – was not significantly associated with depression (Greening & Stoppelbein, 2002; Pearce, Little, & Perez, 2003). Among adolescents, perhaps it is the interpersonal, communal dimension of religious involvement that may attenuate depression.

Religion and Serious Illness

Religion and spirituality has been shown to impact physical health as well. In particular, most research has been done among adolescents who are coping with chronic or serious illness, such as cancer or renal failure. In one sophisticated study, among 114 hospitalized adolescents, the more serious the illness, the more spiritual and religious their concerns were. Further, African-American and female adolescents were more likely to have religious and spiritual concerns (Smith et al., 2002).

One study performed rigorous qualitative interviews with families whose adolescent children were undergoing cancer treatment. Among the 259 patients and their parents, religious and spiritual coping was positively associated with family support and school performance. These researchers also found that that the family's social field narrowed and relationships with close friends strengthened (Spilka 1991). In another study among cancer patients, religious coping and other existential aspects of spirituality were helpful in providing acceptance of one's chronic condition and security in face of death (Tebbi 1987).

RELIGION AND CYSTIC FIBROSIS

An interesting study that has particular importance to specialists who treat complicated patients in collaborative fashion evaluated non-traditional and religious treatments among patients with cystic fibrosis. Stern et al., (1992) found that, among 402 patients with cystic fibrosis, 70% sought non-medical therapy, 60% used "religious treatments" such as prayer, pilgrimage, and possession of religious objects. 92% perceived benefits to these interventions (Stern, Canda, & Doershuk, 1992). This study has important implications to providers – especially for complicated patients. Most patients engage in non-traditional therapies and the vast majority believe they are helpful. It is important that we providers ask about such therapies. What do they entail? Could they be harmful? Do the treatments incite the patient not to follow traditional medical therapy? Could a patient say, "God will heal me so I don't need to take my antibiotics?" Is there a way to incorporate the patient's belief systems in the tertiary care setting that both affirms the patient's beliefs and the importance of evidence-based modern care? These issues are important to pursue.

In another study about children with cystic fibrosis, Pendleton et al., (2002) examined the childrens' spiritual lives as well as their parents. They found three differences. First, children used different spiritual coping strategies than adults such as declarative intervention where the child believes God will intervene in their lives immediately. Second, children reported less negative coping strategies than adults (i.e., blaming God). Third, in keeping with their developmental and cognitive stage, children used less sophisticated forms of spirituality (Pendleton et al., 2002).

LIMITATIONS AND FURTHER QUESTIONS

There are some limitations to the study of religion and spirituality among adolescents. First, there is no gold standard measurement for religion and spirituality among adolescents. Instruments tend to have adult language with adult focus (Cotton 2006). Most studies use attendance and participation in religious activities as their primary marker (Rew & Wong, 2006). Simply measuring attendance is of questionable validity, even among adults. Attendance at worship may be compulsory in some families, thereby masking the true motivations of the adolescent.

Another important question to pursue in exploring the spirituality of adolescents is how one's religious life changes over time? The demographics of church life are very compelling. Children of church-going parents are much more likely to attend church in adulthood (Smith et al., 2002). But how does the spiritual life change over time for an adolescent? Since most studies are cross-sectional, longitudinal studies are needed to follow how spirituality modulates over time.

Further, in an increasingly pluralistic age, there are very few studies outside of the Judeo-Christian tradition that explore how religiosity impacts the health and well-being of adolescents. This is a rich area to explore that includes cross-cultural challenges. Several studies show that religion is more important to the African American community than the Caucasian one – especially during times of stress. 44 But, how religion impacts the life of African Americans and other minority groups can shed light on the richness and complexity of religious expression (Hines 1996). Finally, there are few studies regarding religion and adolescents who are gay, bisexual, or transgendered. Such adolescents may feel ostracized by their religious community.

What does this mean for our adolescent patients? There are real, lasting, serious consequences to the health behaviors of our adolescent patients. More than that, there are great pressures by peer groups to take risk, experiment with drugs, alcohol, and engage in sexual behaviors. Adolescence is an age of increasing autonomy, where increasing independence, in a supportive environment, is critical towards the development of a mature adult. When peer groups have an outsized influence, greater than their parents, religion can play a key role in their development. Religious involvement can provide that important foundation of community support, accountability, and values that allows for autonomous growth for an adolescent.

Our role should be to inquire about the importance of religion in the lives of our adolescent patients, encourage exploration, support them in their choices, but maintain a positive appreciation around the importance of religious involvement. At a time when there can be so little to offer in face of peer pressure and other forces, perhaps religious involvement is one of the few important forces that can make a difference in an adolescent's life.

REFERENCES

Blum, R. W., & Nelson-Mmari, K. (2004). The health of young people in a global context. *Journal of Adolescent Health*, *35*(5), 402-418.

Centers for Disease Control (CDC). (2006). Leading Causes of Death Among Adolescents Aged 15-19, 2006, National Center for Health Statistics, National Vital Statistics System, Retrieved on February 1st, 2016 from: http://mchb.hrsa.gov/chusa08/hstat/hsa/images/50a_08adolescentmortality_causes.gif.

Cotton, S., Larkin, E., Hoopes, A., Cromer, B. A., & Rosenthal, S. L. (2005). The impact of adolescent spirituality on depressive symptoms and health risk behaviors. *Journal of Adolescent Health*, *36*(6), 529.

Cotton, S., Zebracki, K., Rosenthal, S. L., Tsevat, J., Drotar, D., (2006). Religion/spirituality and adolescent health outcomes: a review, *Journal of Adolescent Health.* 38, 472-480

Dalby, J., Hayon, R., & Carlson, J. (2014). Adolescent pregnancy and contraception. *Primary Care: Clinics in Office Practice*, *41*(3), 607-629.

Freedman, D. S., Dietz, W. H., Srinivasan, S. R., & Berenson, G. S. (1999). The relation of overweight to cardiovascular risk factors among children and adolescents: the Bogalusa Heart Study. *Pediatrics*, *103*(6), 1175-1182.

Gallup, G. H., & Bezilla, R. (1992). The religious life of young Americans. *Princeton, NJ: George H. Gallup International Institute*.

Greening, L, Stoppelbein, L. (2002). Religiosity, attributional style, and social support as psychosocial buffers for African American and White adolescents' perceived risk for suicide. Suicide and Life Threatening Behavior 32(4), 404 –17.

Hines, P. M., Boyd-Franklin, N. (1996) Ethnicity and Family Therapy, 2nd ed. New York, NY: Guilford Press.

Hodge, D. R., Cardenas, P., Montoya, H. (2001). Substance use: spirituality and religious participation as protective factors among rural youths. *Social Work Research* 25(3), 153–62.

Holder, D. W., DuRant, R. H., Harris, T. L., Daniel, J. H., Obeidallah, D., & Goodman, E. (2000). The association between adolescent spirituality and voluntary sexual activity. *Journal of adolescent health*, *26*(4), 295-302.

Kessler, R. C., Avenevoli, S., & Merikangas, K. R. (2001). Mood disorders in children and adolescents: an epidemiologic perspective. *Biological psychiatry*, *49*(12), 1002-1014.

Lammers, C., Ireland, M., Resnick, M., Blum, R. (2000). Influences on adolescents' decision to postpone onset of sexual intercourse: a survival analysis of virginity among youths aged 13 to 18 years. *Journal of Adolescent Health*, 26, 42– 8.

Mulye, T. P., Park, M. J., Nelson, C. D., Adams, S. H., Irwin, C. E., & Brindis, C. D. (2009). Trends in adolescent and young adult health in the United States. *Journal of Adolescent Health*, *45*(1), 8-24.

Must, A., & Strauss, R. S. (1999). Risks and consequences of childhood and adolescent obesity. *International Journal of Obesity & Related Metabolic Disorders*, *23*.

Ollendick, T. H., Grills, A. E., & Alexander, K. L. (2001). Fears, worries, and anxiety in children and adolescents. *Anxiety disorders in children and adolescents: Epidemiology, risk factors and treatment*, 1-36.

Pearce, M. J., Little, T. D., & Perez, J. E. (2003). Religiousness and depressive symptoms among adolescents. *Journal of Clinical Child and Adolescent Psychology*, *32*(2), 267-276.

Pendleton, S. M., Cavalli, K. S., Pargament, K. I., & Nasr, S. Z. (2002). Religious/spiritual coping in childhood cystic fibrosis: A qualitative study. *Pediatrics*, *109*(1), e8-e8.

Regnerus, M. D. (2003). Religion and positive adolescent outcomes: A review of research and theory. *Review of Religious Research*, 394-413.

Resnick, M. D., Harris, L. J., Blum, R. W. (1993). The impact of caring and connectedness on adolescent health and well-being. *Journal of Paediatric and Child Health*, 29, S3–9 (suppl 1).

Resnick, M. D., Bearman, P. S., Blum, R. W., Bauman, K. E., Harris, K. M., Jones, J., ... & Ireland, M. (1997). Protecting adolescents from harm: findings from the National Longitudinal Study on Adolescent Health. *Jama*, *278*(10), 823-832.

Rew, L., Thomas, N., Horner, S. D., Resnick, M. D., & Beuhring, T. (2001). Correlates of recent suicide attempts in a triethnic group of adolescents. *Journal of Nursing Scholarship*, *33*(4), 361-367.

Rew, L., & Wong, J. (2006). A systematic review of associations among religiosity/spirituality and adolescent health attitudes and behaviors, *Journal of Adolescent Health*, 38:433-442.

Ritt-Olson, A., Milam, J., Unger, J. B., Trinidad, D., Teran, L., Dent, C. W., & Sussman, S. (2004). The protective influence of spirituality and "health-as-a-value" against monthly substance use among adolescents varying in risk. *Journal of Adolescent Health*, *34*(3), 192-199.

Smith, C., Denton, M. L., Faris, R., & Regnerus, M. (2002). Mapping American adolescent religious participation. *Journal for the Scientific Study of Religion*, 597-612.

Smith, C., Denton, M. L., (2005). Soul Searching: The Religious and Spiritual Lives of American Teenagers. New York, NY: Oxford University Press.

Spilka, B., Zwartjes, W. J., Zwartjes, G. M., (1991). The role of religion in coping with childhood cancer. *Pastoral Psychology*, 39(5), 295–304.

Stern, R. C., Canda, E. R., & Doershuk, C. F. (1992). Use of nonmedical treatment by cystic fibrosis patients. *Journal of Adolescent Health, 13*(7), 612-615.

Tebbi, C. K., Mallon, J. C., Richards, M. E., Bigler, L. R. (1987). Religiosity and locus of control of adolescent cancer patients. *Psychological Reports,* 61(3), 683–96.

Wallace, J. M., Brown, T. N., Bachman, J. G., & LaViest, T. A. (2003). *Religion, race, abstinence from drug use among American adolescents.* Institute for Social Research.

Wallace, J. M., Forman, T. A. (1998). Religion's role in promoting health and reducing risk among American youth [Special issue: public health and health education in faith communities]. Health Education Behavior, 25(6), 721–41.

Wills, T. A., Yaeger, A. M., Sandy, J. M. (2003). Buffering effect of religiosity for adolescent substance use. *Psycholoigy of Addictive Behaviors,* 17(1), 24 –31.

Wright, L. S., Frost, C. J., & Wisecarver, S. J. (1993). Church attendance, meaningfulness of religion, and depressive symptomatology among adolescents. *Journal of Youth and Adolescence*, *22*(5), 559-568.

Chapter 7

Spirituality and the Coping of Chronic Disease

While religion and spirituality impacts overall longevity, mental health, and sense of well-being, coping with chronic illness presents an important challenge for patients and providers alike. Illnesses such as diabetes, hypertension, and chronic back pain are dependent upon a host of factors to their overall successful care - medical compliance, follow up with appointments, and coping with uncertainty. Chronic illness can be particularly frustrating for a patient; diagnoses can be hard to understand and regimens can be complex and frustrating. Resolution of their problems is distant, if possible at all. Success can also be elusive. A person with chronic pain will have good days and bad. The person with diabetes will have good glycemic control some days and poor control others. Patients with chronic illness are more likely to be depressed, have legal and family stress, and face economic hardships. They are also more likely to attempt suicide (Ruoff 1996). Coping with chronic illness requires hope and endurance for the long term. How does religiosity and spirituality impact coping with chronic illness?

Rippentrop et al., (2005) evaluated 122 patients with chronic pain. She found that patients with chronic pain are more likely to feel abandoned by God and feel less desire to reduce pain in the world. Interestingly, private religious practices – such as engaging in prayer or meditation – were inversely correlated with physical health outcomes. The worse the patient felt, the more they engaged in religious practices. She posits that religion and spirituality was an important resource for coping with debilitated health. Experiencing a lack of forgiveness and negative religious coping was also associated with greater pain intensity. A similar relationship was found among 3,851 patients elderly patients. Those who prayed, meditated, or read the Bible daily had greater physical disability than those who engaged in those practices weekly (Haley, Koenig, & Bruchett, 2001).

However, this association has not been replicated in other studies. Turner & Clancy (1986) found that increased hope and prayer was significantly related to decreased pain intensity. Another study by Keefe et al., (2001) studied 35 patients suffering from chronic pain due to rheumatoid arthritis. In an ingenious study, patients were asked to keep a daily diary for 30 consecutive days that addressed spiritual experiences and coping. Keefe et al., (2001) discovered that variability in coping and spiritual experiences was high from day to day. When patients employed spiritual and religious coping strategies well, their pain was much less. Also, patients noted the importance of social support in controlling pain (Keefe et al., 2001).

An important study by Koenig (2002) evaluated religious beliefs among patients with congestive heart failure and chronic pulmonary disease admitted to a tertiary care hospital. Among 196 patients, 98% had a religious affiliation, 48% reported attending religious services weekly or more, and 85% incorporated religious beliefs into their worldview. Religious activities and attitudes were inversely related to physical illness severity and functional disability.

An interesting study among African Americans with hypertension revealed that systolic and diastolic blood pressure was lower among those who attended church frequently (Koenig et al., 1998). Another study among African Americans, this time among women with diabetes, demonstrated improved glycemic control (Newlin et al., 2008). Among patients with multiple sclerosis, McNulty et al., (2004) evaluated 50 patients and showed that spiritual well-being was associated with psychosocial adjustment. These mixed findings suggest the complex relationship between disease and religion. Beliefs fluctuate over time. Coping is better on some days than others. The *quality* of coping seems to have an association: a negative view of God appears to correlate with greater pain, whereas positive coping may correlate with reduced pain.

THE UNIQUE STORY OF HUMAN IMMUNODEFICIENCY VIRUS

In recent years, due to advances made with highly active retrovirus therapy, even HIV infection has moved into the realm of chronic disease. If patients are compliant with their medication regimen, the virus can be suppressed and the immune system rebounds to near normal function. In fact, the care of HIV has moved into a chronic disease model, where we are discovering patients with HIV have higher prevalence of cancer, heart disease, and stroke. The religious lives of patients with HIV are particularly interesting due to the nature of the infection. Intravenous drug use and unprotected homosexual intercourse are topics often difficult to address within religious groups.

In particular, many religious groups see unprotected homosexual intercourse as particularly taboo. However, the church may inflict particular judgment upon those who are infected with HIV through intravenous drug use or unprotected heterosexual intercourse. No matter how a patient acquires HIV infection, they may perceive it as a marker for shameful or sinful activity. As such, HIV is often kept as a private matter by the patient and not shared with one's religious group in the same way as they might if one had cancer or diabetes.

I say all this as a physician who has dedicated a significant portion of his career to the care of patients with HIV. Rosa, the patient described in the first chapter, found great refuge and comfort in the church. But, to date, she has not shared her HIV positive status. There are other stories. One woman acquired HIV from her male partner. She had never used intravenous drugs. Indeed, she was monogamous. Her HIV infection was devastating. Her church was a conservative, traditional urban church where the women wore white dresses and white gloves. Although she is deeply spiritual and attends regularly, she too has not divulged her status and maintains her role as a "proper church lady."

This fear of rejection ostracism goes beyond the community. Many HIV patients feel a sense of divine judgment, that God is punishing them, that they deserve their fate. And so, among this particularly unique population, how does religiosity and spirituality impact the health and wellbeing of HIV patients?

Religion and spirituality is important to patients with HIV. An important study evaluated 2266 patients from the HIV Cost and Utilization Study (HCSUS). 85% responded that spirituality was "somewhat" or "very important" to their lives. 65% identified religion as the same. 72% responded that they "often" or "sometimes" used religion and spirituality when making decisions; and 65% responded that they use religion and spirituality when they confront problems (Lorenz et al., 2005).

And so, religion and spirituality are important to patients with HIV. More than that, many studies have shown that increased religiosity and spirituality is correlated with increased emotional and spiritual wellness. The largest of these studies evaluated 450 patients across four medical centers. Lower spiritual well-being and less social support correlated with worse depression (Yi et al., 2006). In the same way, those patients with greater spirituality and religion scores believed that "life is better now than previously" (Szaflarski et al., 2006).

An important question is how spirituality and religiosity may impact biological outcomes such as HIV viral load and t-cell counts? There are only two studies to date. Perhaps the best is a longitudinal study that followed 100 HIV positive patients over 4 years. Over this time, those patients who increased their religious commitments – through both their belief and attendance had greater preservation of their t-cells and better viral load control (Ironson, Stuetzle, & Fletcher, 2006). Another study among 106 HIV positive gay men showed that religious behavior – such as church attendance – correlated with increased T-cells and CD4 percentage. However, religious coping – a more internal measure regarding prayer and faith in God – did not impact t-cell count (Woods et al., 1999).

Instead of spiritual wellness, Kremer (2015) explored spiritual struggle among HIV infected patients, which included regarding their infection as divine punishment and feeling guilty about their infection. Patients who experienced greater spiritual struggle had worse viral load control and several other worse outcomes. They tended to experience more somatic symptoms – such as chronic pain and fatigue – and attributed them to their HIV infection. Patients with more spiritual struggle also acknowledged a lower quality of life, more depressive symptoms, poorer esteem, and lower social support (Kremer, 2015).

Religiosity, Addiction and Risk Taking Behaviors

Not only health outcomes are improved with religiosity, but also risk-taking behavior. Several studies show that attendance at religious services and religious attitudes are associated with lower rates of alcoholism and binge drinking (Bowie, Ensminger, & Robertson, 2006; Dunn, 2005; Ford & Kadushin, 2002). Religious involvement has also been associated with lower use of other illicit drugs as well (Dunn, 2005; Miller, 1998).

Religiosity has been helpful in prison populations as well. In a study about recidivism, 400 inmates were randomized to a monthly Bible study and compared to a control with no Bible study (Johnson, Larson, & Pitts, 1997). At one year follow up, 14% of the Bible study participants had returned to prison whereas 41% of the control arm had returned to prison. This means that for every 3.7 inmates enrolled in a monthly Bible study, one person stayed out of jail at one year (Johnson, Larson, & Pitts 1997). The implications for this are enormous. What happens in a Bible study that is different from, say, a regular support group? Could it be that a person can place their lives in a greater context of God and community? Could it be that a person can understand a way out of their crime? Their guilt? Their shame? This study raises the question about how real healing occurs. It is not enough to merely "pay one's debt to society" and then re-integrate back into society. I wonder if deeper transformation must occur. People need to change in their core or their external behaviors will not change. Perhaps a Bible study guides that transformation and reveals to a prisoner how they are no longer prisoners to their old ways, to sin, to brokenness. A faith-based intervention may guide an inmate to acknowledge the past, but not have the past define them. Inmates can be guided to see that they are new creations, and that their old ways have no claim to them.

In a similar study that addressed opioid addiction, 248 patients were followed over a 12 year period. 27 patients entered a religious-based treatment program. The others enrolled in conventional, public hospital type treatment. At one year, 45% of patients in the religious treatment arm were still abstinent versus 5% in the standard public hospital treatment (Desmond & Maddux, 1981). The authors note that major improvements in life-style and risk-taking behaviors were noted. This project is particularly powerful because 87% of those addicted where ethnic minorities (Desmond & Maddux, 1981).

Like the recidivism study, this study suggests that there is something unique to a religious-based treatment program. Since these are correlations, the major critique is that of selection bias. Patients needed to consent to enter a religious-based treatment program. Right away, does that confer some advantage? Is there extra motivation or spiritual hunger that nudges a hurting person to seek spiritual care? While this critique is valid. It is valid only partially. Many patients are motivated to seek care, and do so. In the study of Desmond & Maddux (1981), many people entered traditional care but relapsed.

How do we apply this data to the care of our patients? There will always be methodological considerations. And yet, there is something powerful about spirituality and the religious community in particular that supplements conventional care. My own opinion is that the hardest barrier to overcome for engaging in a religious community for a person struggling with addiction is the perceived notion that he will be judged. The addict's shame is projected upon the congregation.

One of my own patients was struggling with addiction. I was treating her with buprenorphine/naltrexone, a partial opioid blocker. And yet, despite earnest attempts at abstinence, she had relapsed several times with heroin. She cited the triggers of "running into my old crowd," and "I got into an argument with my family and getting high was what I am used to doing." When asked about her religious life, she shared that she had a warm association with a church in the neighborhood. But she shared, "They will never accept me. They know too much about me and the things that I've done."

After much conversation, I wrote out a prescription, "Attend church this Sunday." I also asked that she return with the church bulletin – to close an accountability loop. She attended church and showed the minister the prescription that I had written her. Fortunately, she was warmly received and felt a jolt of acceptance that she realized she sorely missed. Only by attending church, did she realize the emptiness in her life and her attempts at filling this emptiness with heroin. Additionally, she recognized a path to wholeness and self-affirmation. What was particularly powerful what that the congregation *did* know all about her past – and accepted her anyway. Since that experience, she has been abstinent from heroin.

The interplay between spirituality, religion and chronic illness is complex. While many studies show a positive association, others are equivocal. Also, in this body of research, the *quality* of religiosity and spiritualty is important. Spiritual struggle, negative religious coping is associated with poorer health outcomes. This points to how complex this field is. Religion and spirituality are part internal belief, social construct, intentional practice and intellectual endeavor. As a healthcare provider exploring these issues with patient can reveal an important resource for coping, hoping, and healing.

References

Bowie, J. V., Ensminger, M. E., & Robertson, J. A. (2006). Alcohol-use problems in young black adults: effects of religiosity, social resources, and mental health. *Journal of Studies on Alcohol*, *67*(1), 44-53.

Desmond, D. P., & Maddux, J. F. (1981). Religious programs and careers of chronic heroin users. *The American journal of drug and alcohol abuse*, *8*(1), 71-83.

Dunn, M. S. (2005). The relationship between religiosity, employment, and political beliefs on substance use among high school seniors. *Journal of Alcohol and Drug Education*, *49*(1), 73.

Ford, J., & Kadushin, C. (2002, June). Between sacral belief and moral community: A multidimensional approach to the relationship between religion and alcohol among whites and blacks. In *Sociological Forum* (Vol. 17, No. 2, pp. 255-279). Kluwer Academic Publishers-Plenum Publishers.

Haley, K. C., Koenig, H. G., & Bruchett, B. M. (2001). Relationship between private religious activity and physical functioning in older adults. *Journal of Religion and Health*, *40*(2), 305-312.

Ironson, G., Stuetzle, R., & Fletcher, M. A. (2006). An increase in religiousness/spirituality occurs after HIV diagnosis and predicts slower disease progression over 4 years in people with HIV. *Journal of General Internal Medicine*, *21*(S5), S62-S68.

Johnson, B. R., Larson, D. B., & Pitts, T. G. (1997). Religious programming, institutional adjustment and recidivism among former inmates in prison fellowship programs. *Justice Quarterly*, 14, 145-166.

Keefe, F. J., Affleck, G., Lefebvre, J., Underwood, L., Caldwell, D. S., Drew, J., et al., (2001). Living with rheumatoid arthritis: The role of daily spirituality and daily religious and spiritual coping. *The Journal of Pain*, *2*(2), 101-110.

Koenig, H. G. (2002). Religion, congestive heart failure, and chronic pulmonary disease. *Journal of Religion and Health*, *41*(3), 263-278.

Koenig, H., George, L. K., Larson, D. B., Cohen, H. J., & Blazer, D. G. (1998). The relationship between religious activities and blood pressure in older adults. *International Journal of Psychiatry in Medicine*, *28*, 189-213.

Kremer, H., Ironson, G., Kaplan, L., Stuetzele, R., Baker, N., & Fletcher, M. A. (2015). Spiritual coping predicts CD4-cell preservation and undetectable viral load over four years. *AIDS Care*, *27*(1), 71-79.

Lorenz, K. A., Hays, R. D., Shapiro, M. F., Cleary, P. D., Asch, S. M., & Wenger, N. S. (2005). Religiousness and spirituality among HIV-infected Americans. *Journal of Palliative Medicine*, *8*(4), 774-781.

McNulty, K., Livneh, H., & Wilson, L. M. (2004). Perceived uncertainty, spiritual well-being, and psychosocial adaptation in individuals with multiple sclerosis. *Rehabilitation Psychology*, *49*(2), 91.

Miller, W. R. (1998). Researching the spiritual dimensions of alcohol and other drug problems. *Addiction*, *93*(7), 979-990.

Newlin, K., Melkus, G. D., Tappen, R., Chyun, D., & Koenig, H. G. (2008). Relationships of religion and spirituality to glycemic control in Black women with type 2 diabetes. *Nursing research*, *57*(5), 331-339.

Rippentrop, A. E., Altmaier, E. M., Chen, J. J., Found, E. M., & Keffala, V. J. (2005). The relationship between religion/spirituality and physical health, mental health, and pain in a chronic pain population. *Pain*, *116*(3), 311-321.

Ruoff, G. E. (1996). Depression in the patient with chronic pain. *Journal of Family Practice*, *43*(6), S25-S25.

Szaflarski, M., Neal Ritchey, P., Leonard, A. C., Mrus, J. M., Peterman, A. H., Ellison, C. G., McCullough, M. E., & Tsevat, J. (2006). Modeling the effects of spirituality/religion on patients' perceptions of living with HIV/AIDS. *Journal of General Internal Medicine*, *21*(S5), S28-S38.

Turner, J. A., & Clancy, S. (1986). Strategies for coping with chronic low back pain: relationship to pain and disability. *Pain*, *24*(3), 355-364.

Yi, M. S., Mrus, J. M., Wade, T. J., Ho, M. L., Hornung, R. W., Cotton, S., ... & Tsevat, J. (2006). Religion, spirituality, and depressive symptoms in patients with HIV/AIDS. *Journal of General Internal Medicine*, *21*(S5), S21-S27.

Chapter 8

HEALTH AND HEALING AMONG NON-CHRISTIANS

In the 2015 Gallup poll, 77% of the population identified themselves as being Christian (Gallup 2015). This reveals a significant population that is non-Christian. And American society becomes increasing diverse. By the year 2042, whites will no longer be the majority of the population, which will then include people of African, Latino, and Asian descent (Craig 2014). This represents a particular challenge to the healthcare provider who seeks sensitive care towards those of a religious group different from mainstream society. For this reason, in recent years, cultural competence has become an important part of medical school and residency program curriculum.

But is cultural competence enough? What is "cultural competence" exactly? An important aspect of cultural competence is *curiosity*. We must be curious, interested in, open to the perspective of another religion. It is impossible to lump the entire Christian world into a coherent set of beliefs. Indeed, wars have been fought over such beliefs. In the same way, it is impossible to assume that all Muslims (or Hindus or Jews for that matter) adhere to same beliefs. A provider might ask, "You have shared with me that you are a practicing Muslim, what aspects of your religion are important to you as we think about your new cancer diagnosis?" This open-ended question invites further dialogue.

It is important to consider that not "all religions are the same." This is as offensive as saying, "All white people are the same," or, "All Americans are the same." To lump all religions together is to do disservice to them all. Each has a rich perspective, a unique worldview, a powerful claim on truth. Different religions may, in fact, look more similar in their particularity and quite different in their core beliefs. Each religion has some form of priesthood – a separate group of specialists who lead or guide the people. They almost always wear special vestments or have titles that separate them from the rest of society. Each group has some liturgy or rites that entail people gathering together to worship.

And yet, the core beliefs of each religion – and even within religious sects – are quite different. Regarding the divinity of Jesus, C.S. Lewis famously wrote, "There is no half-way house, and there is no parallel in other religions. If you had gone to Buddha and asked him, 'Are you the son of Brahah?' he would have said, 'My son, you are still in the vale of illusion.' If you had gone to Socrates and asked, 'Are you Zeus?' he would have laughed at you. If you had gone to Muhammad and asked, 'Are you Allah?' he would first have rent his clothes and then cut off your head' " (Lewis, 2014).

In the West, God is a Being separate from the self. We pray *to* God. God is *other*. We commune with God, have a relationship with God. In the East, God is *One*. God is *within*. God is *all*. This is the difference between monadism (God is one, but other) and monisim (God is one, in all). While this appears like an academic difference, the implications of this belief affect healing and disease. While each religion is different, they do not disagree. Each religion reflects a certain worldview born from cultural influences, history, scripture, and economics. For thousands of years, each religion has evolved independently from each other. Only in recent centuries have real cross fertilization taken place. This inter-relationship has only increased in recent decades.

I write this chapter as a Christian who is curious about the religious and spiritual life of my patients. As such, I seek to address the question, "How does the religious perspective of your religion impact your understanding of health?" I do not pretend to be an expert in these various traditions. Instead, I seek out the voices of others who are. I find that each religion has its own language. Each word - tao, karma, sin, grace - has its own history and context that the believer registers. It can be difficult for an outsider to really understand the cultural significance and the spiritual resonance of such words. The Bhagavad Gita is an important scripture for Hindus, but to call it the "Hindu Bible" is not entirely accurate either.

This richness of belief is one reason that being a clinician is so wonderful. Our patients' health can be the lens by which we understand another's religion and culture, bewildering to us as it may be. The other dimension to understanding the religious beliefs of a minority religion is the very identity as a "minority." Islam may feel different to a believer in Baghdad, Iraq when compared to Asheville, North Carolina. Hinduism may have a different feel in New Delhi, India than in Schenectady, New York. The very self-identity as a religious minority may impact their religious experience.

Further, while there are various traditions within each religion, the individual patient may or may not adhere to all the tenets of their faith. There are Catholics who have no trouble with birth control; and Jehovah's Witnesses who allow blood transfusions when it can save the life of their children. And so, to cast a patient as a Hindu, Muslim, Buddhist, or Jew does not mean that the practitioner will understand their worldview any more than knowing that their patient is a Christian. Intensity and orthodoxy of belief, of course, varies quite widely among individuals.

At the very same time, to attempt some generalization, in broad strokes, of the general principles of Islam, Hinduism, Buddhism and Judaism can be helpful in understanding the world view of our patients. I approach this topic with humility. These are grand traditions with centuries of tradition, rich sacred literature, highly developed intellectual traditions, and a diversity of expression. Thus, there is no unifying paradigm to identify any singular tradition. In seems, as soon as you lay claim to the primacy of one doctrine, there is a significant branch that takes issue. For example, the primacy of the Virgin Mary is quite different between Catholicism and Protestantism. I apologize in advance for distilling the richness of these traditions into a few brief paragraphs. As we consider the beliefs of those who may be different from the majority American religion, the question becomes: *what is it about my patient's particular religion that impacts their health?* What do I need to understand to treat patients who may have a different perspective with respect, understanding, and compassion?

HEALTH AND ISLAM

Islam has a rich and storied history in the development of modern medicine. Large and sophisticated hospitals were developed in the Muslim world hundreds of years before Europe. Hospitals were built in Damascus, Syria in 706CE, Baghdad, Iraq in 750CE, and Cairo, Egypt in 872CE. One of the greatest hospitals – the Mansuri – in Cairo was founded in 1284 CE and accommodated 8,000 people. The large staff included surgeons and physicians, a complex administration, and sophisticated teaching facilities. In a very real way, the Mansuri was the forerunner of the modern academic medical center (Nagamia 2003). Of course, the hero of Islamic medicine is Ibn

Sina, whose name is often Latinized to Avicenna. His eminent work, *The Canon of Medicine*, based on Aristotelian principles of logic, comprised more than 14 volumes addressed every aspect of medicine known at the time. Initially published in 1025, this work was transmitted to Europe and formed the backbone of medical education from the 12th to the 17th century (Smith 1980).

There are approximately 1.3 billion Muslims in the world, making it the second largest religion behind Christianity. 25% live in the Indian subcontinent, 20% in sub-Saharan Africa, 17% in Southeast Asia, 18% in the Arab world, 10% in the republics of the old Soviet Union and China, 10% in the non-Arab middle East. There are approximately 7-8 million Muslims in the United States comprising 1-2% of the population (Johnson, 2013).

The word "Islam" simply means "submission," and also derives from the word meaning "peace." (Rassool 2000) There are five core articles of faith in Islam, which foster connectedness with God:

1. Tawhid or belief in the Oneness of Allah – This is the fundamental teaching of Islam. Islam shares the belief with Christianity that the prophets of the Hebrew Scripture - beginning with Adam and including Abraham, Isaac, Jacob, and Moses. Jesus, too, is considered a prophet. The prophet Muhammad was the last and greatest of the prophets. The scriptures of Judaism and Christianity are considered to connote revealed truth, but the Qu'ran completes and supersedes all previous revelations. The word for God – Allah – is used by Muslims and Christians alike in the Middle East.
2. Salat or contractual prayer – these obligatory prayers are designated 5 times a day. There is a direct link between the worshipper and Allah.
3. Siyam or fasting. During the month of Ramadhan, Muslims fast from sunrise to sunset, abstaining from all eating, drinking, and sexual relations. In addition to the fast, there are increased prayers and exercises of mindfulness, having positive thoughts towards others and God, in all thoughts and actions.
4. Zakah - Often translated as charity, the concept of Zakah also means purification and growth. Our wealth is held in trust by human beings. Our possessions, then, are purified, made holy, by giving a proportion to the poor. As the prophet Muhammad proclaimed, "The wealth of a servant is never decreased by paying charity."
5. Hajj or pilgrimage to Mecca in Saudi Arabia. This is an obligation for all Muslims once in a lifetime, unless physically or financially unable.

Worshippers wear a simple garment which strips away social status, country, and color, so that all are united in the human community and stand equal before God (Rassool 2000, Syed 2003).

These core beliefs lead to a holistic understanding of the person, the community, and the Oneness of God. Thus, suffering and illness has a physical, spiritual, and social importance. The consequences of these core beliefs have significant positive impact upon one's mental and emotional health. Syed (2003) points out that the "contact prayer- a remembrance of Allah and corporate worship - by itself fosters a richness and connectivity. He cites the Qu'ran, "Worship in the congregation is more excellent than Worship alone, by twenty seven degrees." Both the Hajj and the commitment to corporate worship gives community and meaning to the believer. He cites the physiologic responses of relaxation and contentment that it developed with the important practice of regular prayer 5 times a day. Fasting, too, has several positive effects including improved mood and bodily functions (Syed, 2003). The principle of *zakah*, or practicing charity, is also an important principle that enriches both community bonds and also affirms the importance of empathy and living outside oneself. This perspective has also been shown to have positive mental health benefits (Syed, 2003).

Like Christianity, there is a high regard for the Islamic sacred scripture, the Qur'an. The Qur'an is believed to be the direct revelation of God to the prophet Mohammed as revealed by the angel Gabriel. Syed (2003) cites the tradition of "miraculous properties" of the Qur'an whereby certain passages are believed to carry curative powers. For example, one tradition holds that if Surah 38 (also called Surah Sad after the 18th letter in the Arabic alphabet) is recited over a sleeping person, it will cure breathing problems. When written down and read during a patient's waking hours, it cures illness. A person who continuously recites the passage will be immune from all troubles at night.

Even in the 14th century, the benefits of corporate worship were affirmed. Al-Dhahabi noted that ritual prayer where various body postures are exercised have spiritual, psychological, physical, and moral benefits. Corporate prayer causes "recovery from pain of the heart, stomach, and intestines," produces happiness, suppresses anxiety, and strengthens the body (Syed 2003).

The Muslim worldview towards health is to receive illness with patience, meditation, and prayer. Many Muslims believe that illness is an atonement for one's sins, a test from Allah; and death is a part of a journey to meet God (Rassool 2000). The Qur'an promotes health in 3 ways: the legal approach, the guiding approach, and the direct healing approach. First, the Qur'an makes prescriptions about healthy living: no alcohol or tobacco use, moderate eating, and regular exercise. The Muslim dietary law echoes that followed by Orthodox Jews: no eating of pork or pork products, meat from dead animals, or blood. Second, the guiding approach promotes a healthy and balanced lifestyle as a religious obligation, such as eating wholesome food, living a healthy lifestyle. Third, the "direct healing" approach conveys the healing properties of scripture.

It is important when caring for our patients to have a sense of the holistic nature of Muslim belief. Healthy living is a religious obligation as much as practicing charity and 5-times daily prayer. Thus, it would be incongruent within a Muslim belief system to receive care in a modern, empiric-based medical system without a religious dimension to his care. The physical, the spiritual, the communal, all are interconnected. From the Qur'an, "O mankind we have created you male and female, and have made you into nations and tribes so that you may know each other. Lo! The noblest of you in the sight of Allah is the one with the pious" (Al-Hujurat 49:13).

What does the data show? There are some important studies that demonstrate healthful benefits between Islamic belief and health. Among a group of 244 Muslim college students, religiosity was associated with physical health, mental health, happiness, satisfaction with life, and optimism (Abdel-Kalek 2007). In another study, Muslim religiosity accounted for 15% of the variance in happiness and 60% variance for mental health (Abdel-Kalek 2006). An important study that evaluated Islamic religiosity among 2,909 subjects showed a strong correlation with Islamic religiosity and subjective well-being. This association is unaffected by health deficiencies (Tiliouine 2009). In a study among 6,339 Muslim Kuwaiti adolescents, religiosity was positively correlated with happiness, mental health, and physical health and negatively correlated with anxiety and depression (Abdel-Khalek 2007b). One study among 325 Muslim immigrants in North America showed that religiosity was positively related to fewer psychosomatic symptoms, more happiness in life, and greater job satisfaction (Jamal & Badawi, 1993). Another study among 223 Muslim Kuwaitis found that increased religious commitment correlated with lower systolic and diastolic blood pressures (Al-Kandari 2003).

In the United States, there is often suspicion of Muslims, given recent political events. Our Muslim patients may dress differently and may have non-Western customs. While certain extremist Muslim groups have perhaps propagated a negative stereotype in the West, the average Muslim is less concerned with religious doctrine and more concerned with family, relationships, and financial stability (Tessler 2003). Also, Muslims in the East have democratic aspirations and often see the West as an ally (Inglehart 2003). It is important to affirm that Islam is a religion of compassion and mercy. The earliest hospitals in the world cared for all patients, Muslim and non-Muslim alike, without charge and without judgment. This grand tradition extends from both scripture and tradition.

HEALTH AND HINDUISM

Hinduism is the third largest religious tradition in the world, behind Christianity and Islam, with more than 900 million practitioners. Most live in the Indian subcontinent and Bali. 2% live outside India with 1.5 million in the United States (Johnson, 2013). The very notion of Hinduism being a "religion" is controversial. In the Western tradition, for the most part, religion is a codified set of beliefs based upon the teachings of a central religion figure. The nearest term to "religion" might be "Dharma." Hinduism is "a mixture of cosmic order, sacred law and religious duty." (Wig 1999) Further, the concept of God is very different between the East and the West. In the West, God is the Creator and stands outside of creation. Christians pray to God. In the East, God *is* Creation. Creation is an extension of God. It is the subtle but real difference between monotheism (one God) and monism (God is one). Monism denies the duality of between God and creation. God is Creation. Creation is God. Because of this, there is the famous Sanskrit saying, "God is one but men call him by many names." Not all faith traditions can make that same claim.

After graduation from medical school, I served in south India in a small hospital. It was quite common to see small shrines to the various Hindu deities in a town square, in the front dashboard of a taxi - Vishnu the Protector, Ganesh the elephant god. Among those shrines, it was quite common to see one for Jesus Christ. This perspective influences the Hindu worldview in several ways. First, the Hindu perspective is spiritual and idealistic. Almost all schools of Hinduism claim that true reality is ultimately a spiritual one. There are some central themes to the Hindu worldview. The first is the concept of *attachment*, which is when we are too involved in the world. We desire things we do not have and cling to things we do. Second is *detachment* – the turning away from our physical yearnings and moving towards an ultimate spiritual reality. Third, there is *dharma*, which is the guideline for living one's life. Fourth, there is the principle of *karma*, which governs the unfolding of events based upon the integrity and virtue by which one has lived previous lives.

Fifth, there is *moksha,* which is the release from the cycle of rebirth. Sixth, there is samsara, the process of successive rebirths until one has achieved complete release, *moksha* (Whitman 2007).

The project of Hinduism is to live with integrity, cause no harm, and progress further on the spiritual path according to *dharma*, fulfilling one's sacred duty. The main project is to become detached from the over-involvement of the world, which is material, illusory, and temporary, and turn towards God, a transcendent, immanent, ultimate being. This concept of detachment is shared, and in some ways, amplified by Buddhism which evolved from Hindu practices in India (Whitman 2007). Suffering, for the Hindu, is the unfolding of karma – the direct consequence of past inappropriate action in one's current or past life. Suffering is not so much a punishment as the natural consequence of cosmic moral law. As Whitman (2007) explains, "If a Hindu were to ask 'why me' or feel her circumstances were 'not fair,' a response would be that her current situation is the exactly correct situation for her to be in, given her soul's previous action."

The Bhagavad-Gita states, "Contacts with matter make us feel heat and cold, pleasure and pain.... You must learn to endure fleeing things – they come and go! When these cannot torment a man, when suffering and joy are equal for him and he has courage, he is fit for immortality." (Miller, 2088) When one has achieved detachment, although the body may feel pain, there is no true suffering of the self. Enduring suffering satisfies the cosmic debt for past negative or wrong behavior. Further, pain does not affect the true inner self, only one's physical existence. Thus, our Hindu patients may take comfort in that their suffering has cosmic significance, will aid them on their journey, is part of the unfolding of their place in the universe, and can lead towards the spiritual path towards enlightenment.

When confronting suffering, the Hindu seeks to fulfill one's *dharma*, one purpose, one's duty. Neither is the Hindu to refrain from suffering nor be blindly accepting of suffering. Rather, the project is to accept suffering, strive for detachment, and be mindful of God, the Ultimate. Prayer and other religious practices can be helpful by asking for support, guidance, and acceptance. Central to this belief is the notion of *bhakti* – the concept that God, the Ultimate One, is accessible, knowable, and immanent in personal terms.

For the provider, what are we to do– especially if the concepts of Hinduism are foreign to us? We can encourage connection to the richness of their religious community. While one's *dharma* may lead to an acceptance of illness, some posit that a passivity or fatalism may arise. Our patient's suffering is due to the cosmic law of the universe to pay a debt for past sins.

This can be a heavy burden to bear. The counter to this fatalism is the idea that one can practice right action as a response to suffering. This is different than despondence or despair. Rather, it is a confident acceptance, an acceptance turned towards a cosmic purpose that can bring comfort to suffering. Also, one's *dharma* would include quitting efforts that are ineffective and pursing those practices that can yield effective outcomes (Whitman 2007). With sensitivity and care, the provider can explore a patient's beliefs that may connect him to a supportive community and a healing perspective.

HEALTH AND BUDDHISM

Buddhism is practices by approximately 488-535 million people in the world, accounting for 7-8% of the world's population. China is the country with the most Buddhists, with approximately 244 million or 18.2% of the population. In the United States, there are approximately 3.7 million Buddhists or 1.2% of the population (Johnson, 2013). Like Hinduism, many argue that Buddhism is not truly a religion but rather is a philosophy or even a lifestyle. It is non-theist. Given that there is a coherent worldview, sacred scripture, and community involvement, for the purposes of this work, Buddhism can be understood as a religion.

Buddhism evolved out of the north Indian subcontinent in the 6th BCE as a constellation of teachings, traditions, and beliefs. Siddhartha Gautama, a nobleman and warrior, is credited as discovering a "middle way" - a path that is neither ascetical nor self-indulgent – as a core belief. Siddhartha Gautama became the Buddha, or enlightened one, in a moment of revelation beneath a Bodhi tree in Bodh Gaya, India, where pilgrims continue to visit today (Ratanakul, 2004).

In Buddhism, there are the four noble truths. The first is the truth of *dukkha* which is roughly translated as suffering, anxiety, or unease. Suffering can be physical. We grow old and die. Our suffering can be emotional, from trying to cling to things that are always changing. We are impermanent. The second truth is that the origin of suffering is craving. It is our attachment to this world, to our possessions, to our lives, to our feelings that cause our suffering. At a deeper level, our suffering is caused by our ignorance of the true nature of things, which are largely spiritual. The third truth is that we have the capacity to end our suffering. The fourth noble truth identifies the path to this cessation, which is the Eightfold Path (Ratanakul, 2004).

The Eightfold path consists of an interconnected practice of wisdom (right view and right intention), ethical conduct (right speech, right action, right livelihood), and concentration (right effort, right mindfulness, and right concentration). The central project of the Buddhism worldview is to renounce one's attachment and embrace the true spiritual reality of existence which is the cessation of craving or extinction of ignorance, which has been variously termed *awakening*, *enlightenment*, or *nirvana.* An important feature to one's religious experience is the Middle Way, which is a practice of non-extremism, where the Buddhist neither practices extreme self-mortification or self-indulgence (Ratanakul, 2004). Ratanakul (2004) writes, "The Buddhist holistic perspective... focuses on the whole person and argues that since human beings are not merely physical creatures but mental, emotional, social and spiritual beings as well and that, as a psychosomatic unity, bodily illness affects the mind and emotions and emotional, mental and social maladjustments can affect the body, then to be concerned about a person's health one must be concerned about his entire person, body, mind and emotions, as well as his social environment."

While in the East, medicine and religion has a long symbiotic relationship, in the West, one of the first forays of religion and medicine has been the study of Buddhist meditation. Weaver et al., (2008) performed a systematic review of the literature between 1980 - 2003. He showed that journals publishing topics on Buddhism – meditation in particular – has increased over the decades. Further, scholars who study Buddhism and the journals in which they have published have become increasingly diverse. Instead of only studying Buddhist populations in the East, Western researchers study a wide range of lay and monastic practitioners and their impact on emotional and physical health. Weaver et al., (2008) point out that, in the West, religion and medicine "have warily circled each other since the time of Freud, their suspicions are slowly dissolving in the swirling integrating dance of Eastern and Western thought. Also, there is an emerging interest by Western researchers on the intersection between Buddhist practices and psychological outcomes (Weaver, Vane, & Flannelly, 2008).

Most of the studies that Weaver et al., (2008) highlight address the impact of meditation on emotional and spiritual health. Benson et al., (1990), the Harvard cardiologist, was among the first to study Buddhist monks who showed marked brain wave changes during meditation. Higuchi et al., (1998) studied the impact of Soto Zen priests. After a 40 minute meditation session, the priests showed increased CD4 levels, suggesting improved immune function. Weaver et al., (2008) point out that the word "meditation" is as non-specific catch-all phrase that does disservice to the differences and diversity of different meditation practices. Weaver (2008) writes, "Meditation as a catch all phrase to describe various Buddhist practices is as limiting to our understanding a using the word 'sports' to describe soccer, basketball, and tennis."

In recent years, the Buddhist practice of "mindfulness" had attracted attention. Mindfulness is a "detached observance of one's mental functioning and environments. Sincere dedication to this form my lead a practitioner to experience one-pointedness or nirvana, a place of clear awareness and true insight where the ultimate nature of reality is realized" (Weaver et al., 2008).

Mindfulness has been shown to be a very effective technique towards ameliorating a host of physical and psychologist illness. In one of the more comprehensive studies, 136 patients with a wide range of chronic medical problems were taught to practice mindfulness 20 minutes a day for an 8 week period (Reibel et al., 2001). They then were evaluated with a variety of psychological and physical symptom validated surveys. At the end of the 8 weeks, they showed a significant improvement in their physical symptoms, bodily pain, vitality, and a significant decrease in their pain symptoms. The most dramatic effects were the 44% reduction in anxiety, 38% reduction in global severity, a measure of overall well-being, and a 34% reduction in depressive symptoms. The effect were not just in psychological state. The exercise also improved vitality by 30% and sense of overall physical health by 33%. At one year of follow up, these effects remained statistically significant (Reibel et al., 2001).

Another important meta-analysis collated 1,605 subjects from 64 studies. The patients were afflicted with a wide variety of illnesses including cancer, coronary artery disease, depression, and anxiety. They were randomized to receive mindfulness training. Both mental health and physical health symptoms were improved with mindfulness (Grossman 2004).

In an important longitudinal study, Davidson et al., (2003) studied 25 subjects who were taught mindfulness practices over 8 weeks. They were compared with 16 controls who were wait-listed for the practice. Both electrical activity and immune response was tested. In the intervention group, they showed a heightened left-sided anterior activation, a pattern associated with positive affect. Further, at the end of the 8 weeks, both groups received an influenza vaccine. Those in the meditation group had a heightened antibody titer when compared with the control group. The researchers suggest that even short term meditation can have demonstrable effects in brain activity and immune response (Davidson et al., 2003).

HEALTH AND JUDAISM

Judaism is one of three Abrahamic faiths, along with Christianity and Islam. The Pew Research Center (2012) estimates there are 14 million Jews in the world, 0.2% of the population. Nearly 40% live in the Middle East, almost all in Israel. In the United States, Jews account for more than 5 million or 1.7% of the population. (Pew, 2012) The Jewish approach to healing is based on the Jewish Law (Halacha) which means literally, "the way." (Goldsand, Rosenberg, & Gordon, 2001) While Judaism's core beliefs are the same across the three main traditions – Reform, Conservative, and Orthodox branches – there are significant differences are in the degree of observance (Clarfield et al., 2003).

Jewish practices have had a direct impact upon health in several important studies. Friedlander et al., (1985) compared secular and practicing Jews in Jerusalem. Controlling for demographics, he found that secular persons had a higher prevalence of smoking and higher lipids. These differences were attributed, in part, to the adherence to kosher dietary laws, such as eating kosher meat and avoiding dairy products concurrently or after meat consumption. Observant Jews also had a lower risk of myocardial infarction, perhaps due to the dietary laws (Syder et al., 1978, Friedlander, Kark, & Stein, 1986).

Kark et al., (1996) compared mortality between secular and religious residents of religious communities – Kibbutzim. This study was particularly ingenious since the kibbutzim (plural for kibbutz) have similar social and economic support structures – thereby controlling for much of the social function often attributed as the important factor for health differences between religious and non religious populations. Kark et al., (1996) followed 11 secular and 11 religious kibbutzim for 16 years and found that all cause mortality was considerably higher among the secular communities.

When comparing mortality based on census data in Israel, two cities with high proportions of ultra-orthodox Jews - Jerusalm and Bnei Brak – had the lowest adjusted death rate, despite having lower average incomes (Shemesh & Elkana, 2000). Shmueli & Tamir (2007) did a phone survey among 3,056 urban Israeli Jews. He found that religious Jews had lower prevalence of stress and smoking, but were more obese than secular Jews. Religious Jews followed a healthier diet, but women were less likely to receive mammograms and exercise as secular Jews. There was no difference in religiosity and medical checkups. Religiosity was also positively correlated with happiness among a cohort of Jewish undergraduates (Francis et al., 2004).

As an Abrahamic faith, Judaism shares a similar perspective of God, community, scripture and health as Christianity and Islam. And yet, to assume understanding of Judaism because of a shared religious foundation would be a mistake. Like any religion, there are powerful cultural forces and social norms. There is a distinct intellectual heritage – the Talmud – that gives shape to a Judaic perspective that is unique among all religions. These traditions and distinct perspective give shape to an important understanding of wellness and healing.

THE "NONES" AND HEALTH

By far the largest "religious" minority are the "nones,"- those who self identify as being non-religious - which comprise between 16%-20% of the population (Pew, 2012). This is also the fastest growing segment of the religious landscape in America. This group tends to be younger than those who identify with a faith tradition. 72% are under age 50, compared to 56% of the general public. They tend to be unmarried, have slightly higher levels of income and education (Pew, 2002). This does not mean that religion should not be addressed with such patients. As the data show, there are benefits to practicing one's faith in nearly every realm of medicine – from chronic disease to mental health to cancer and HIV. Importantly, their lack of religious identity does not mean such patients are superficial or lack a spiritual perspective on the world. Many place a high value on relationships and pragmatic values. Much of the language that the non-religious use would resonate with established religion. During time of illness, when facing suffering or death of a loved one or themselves, can be the opportunity of asking questions, doubting, pondering challenging questions. Every belief has a relational component. No belief is static. Dialogue and thoughtful inquire is part of the journey of illness and healing.

How is the provider to respond? Would encouragement be interpreted as proselytization? Would raising a religious issue be received with offensive? I find this question odd. In the clinic, we routinely ask patients about their drug use, their sexual practices, and their alcohol consumption. We examine prostates and vaginas – probing literally the recesses of their bodies. And yet, we are uncomfortable mentioning a proven intervention that may prolong life?

I think the process is best served when it is normalized. It does not seem intrusive to ask, "I know that you have mentioned you are not practicing any religion. One question I ask everyone who struggles with addiction is if they have thought about exploring their religious faith. There is good data to suggest it can help. Have you thought about exploring a religion?" If the answer is no, then a follow up question might be simply, "Why not?" As we know, patients carry all sorts of emotional baggage. Would they feel judged? Was religion too boring as s child? Were they not raised in a faith tradition? We practitioners tend to label our patients too swiftly. Everyone believes in something. These beliefs form the foundation upon how a patient views disease and healing. Further, everyone's beliefs are in some degree of evolution and flux – from the devout Christian to the most ardent atheist. Exploring these issues as it relates to health informs our understanding of our patients' struggles.

CONCLUSION

Perhaps one of the greatest joys in healthcare is connecting around the personal story of our patients. In what other vocation would we encounter such diverse people from such different backgrounds? Medicine is a common bond that unites all people from all backgrounds. Whether our perspective on God or the Holy Scripture we read is different from our patient, this provides an opportunity to learn, to grow, to expand our own worldview. The Muslim has much to teach the Christian about the discipline of prayer. The East has much to teach the West about who God is. Is God one? Is God other? Those who profess no religious affiliation give us a lens to our own doubts. We must be authentic in our own faith – with our own hang-ups and biases – in order to engage honestly with the faith of another. As providers, we must be curious about our patients' faith – as we are curious about all aspects of their culture and life. While all religions are not the same, the *importance* of religion often is in our patients' lives. Engaging the conversation - "How does your religion help you?" – can open doors to coping and healing. "I am not of your religion, and so tell me more about your beliefs?" Honest dialogue and sincere curiosity builds a bond of care between the patient and the provider. This diversity in our patients opens our own understanding and can invigorate our own faith journey.

References

Abdel-Khalek, A. M. (2006). Happiness, health, and religiosity: Significant relations. Mental Health. Religion and Culture, 9(1), 85–97.

Abdel-Khalek, A. M., & Naceur, F. (2007). Religiosity and its association with positive and negative emotions among college students from Algeria. Mental Health, Religion and Culture, 10(2), 159–170.

Abdel-Khalek AM (2007b), Religiosity, happiness, health, and psychopathology in a probability sample of Muslim adolescents, Mental Health, Religion, and Culture, 10(6):571-583.

Al-Kandari, Y. Y. (2003). Religiosity and its relation to blood pressure among selected Kuwaitis. *Journal of Biosocial Science*, 35, 463–472.

Benson, H., Malhotra, M. S., Goldman, R. F., Jacobs, G. D., & Hopkins, P. J. (1990). Three case reports of the metabolic and electroencephalographic changes during advanced Buddhist meditation techniques. *Behavioral Medicine*, *16*(2), 90-95.

Clarfield, A. M., Gordon, M., Markwell, H., & Alibhai, S. M. (2003). Ethical Issues in End-of-Life Geriatric Care: The Approach of Three Monotheistic Religions—Judaism, Catholicism, and Islam. *Journal of the American Geriatrics Society*, *51*(8), 1149-1154.

Craig, M. A., & Richeson, J. A. (2014). On the precipice of a "Majority-Minority" America perceived status threat from the racial demographic shift affects white Americans' political ideology. *Psychological science*, 25, 6:1189-1197.

Davidson, R. J., Kabat-Zinn, J., Schumacher, J., Rosenkranz, M., Muller, D., Santorelli, S. F., ... & Sheridan, J. F. (2003). Alterations in brain and immune function produced by mindfulness meditation. *Psychosomatic medicine*, *65*(4), 564-570.

Francis, L. J., Katz, Y. J., Yablon, Y., & Robbins, M. (2004). Religiosity, personality, and happiness: A study among Israeli male undergraduates. *Journal of Happiness Studies*, *5*(4), 315-333.

Gallup. (2015). Religion. Retrieved February 10th, 2016 from http://www.gallup.com/poll/1690/religion.aspx.

Friedlander, Y., Kark, J. D., Kaufmann, N. A., & Stein, Y. (1985). Coronary heart disease risk factors among religious groupings in a Jewish population sample in Jerusalem. *The American journal of clinical nutrition*, *42*(3), 511-521.

Friedlander, Y., Kark, J. D., & Stein, Y. (1986). Religious orthodoxy and myocardial infarction in Jerusalem—a case control study. *International journal of cardiology*, *10*(1), 33-41.

Goldsand, G., Rosenberg, Z. R., & Gordon, M. (2001). Bioethics for clinicians: 22. Jewish bioethics. *Canadian Medical Association Journal*, *164*(2), 219-222.

Grossman, P., Niemann, L., Schmidt, S., & Walach, H. (2004). Mindfulness-based stress reduction and health benefits: A meta-analysis. *Journal of psychosomatic research*, *57*(1), 35-43.

Higuchi, Y., Kotani, Y., Higuchi, H., & Minegishi, Y. (1998). Immune capability changes during zazen. *Journal of International Society of Life Information Science*, 16, 46–47.

Inglehart, R., & Norris, P. (2003, March/April). The true clash of civilizations. *Foreign Policy*, 135, 67–75.

Jamal, M., & Badawi, J. (1993). Job stress among Muslim immigrants in North America: Moderating effects of religiosity. *Stress Medicine*, 9, 145–151.

Johnson, Todd M.; Grim, Brian J. (2013). *The World's Religions in Figures: An Introduction to International Religious Demography*. Hoboken, NJ: Wiley-Blackwell. pp. 34–37.

Kark, J. D., Shemi, G., Friedlander, Y., Martin, O., Manor, O., & Blondheim, S. H. (1996). Does religious observance promote health? Mortality in secular vs religious kibbutzim in Israel. *American Journal of Public Health*, *86*(3), 341-346.

Lewis, C. S. (2014). *God in the Dock*. Grand Rapids, MI: Wm. B. Eerdmans Publishing.

Miller, B. S. (1988). The Bhagavad-Gita (translation). New York, NY: Bantam Books.

Nagamia, H. F. (2003). Islamic medicine history and current practice. *Journal of the International Society for the history of Islamic medicine*, 2, 19-30.

Pew Research Center, (2012 December 15). The Global Religious Landscape, December 18th, 2012, Retrieved on April 15th, 2015 from, http://www.pewforum.org/2012/12/18/global-religious-landscape-exec/

Rassool, G. H. (2000). The crescent and Islam: healing, nursing and the spiritual dimension. Some considerations towards an understanding of the Islamic perspectives on caring. *Journal of advanced nursing*, *32*(6), 1476-1484.

Ratanakul P. (2004) Buddhism, Health and Disease, *Eubios Journal of Asian and International Bioethics* 15, 162-4.

Reibel, D. K., Greeson, J. M., Brainard, G. C., & Rosenzweig, S. (2001). Mindfulness-based stress reduction and health-related quality of life in a heterogeneous patient population. *General hospital psychiatry*, *23*(4), 183-192.

Smith, R. D. (1980). Avicenna and the Canon of Medicine: a millennial tribute. *Western Journal of Medicine*, *133*(4), 367.

Shemesh, A., & Elkana, Y. (2000). Adjusted Mortality Rates and Socio-Economic Indices in Israeli Localities. *Jerusaelm: Ministry of Health (Hebrew)*.

Shmueli, A., & Tamir, D. (2007). Health behavior and religiosity among Israeli Jews. *The Israel Medical Association journal: IMAJ*, *9*(10), 703-707.

Snyder, M., Goldbourt, U., Medalie, J. H., Neufeld, H. N., & Oron, D. (1978). A lower incidence of myocardial infarction among religious Jews than among irreligious Jews. *Torah Mada*, 8:35–44.

Syed, I. B. (2003). Spiritual medicine in the history of Islamic medicine. *Journal of International Society for the History of Islamic Medicine—JISHAM*, *2*, 45-49.

Tiliouine, H., Cummins, R. A., & Davern, M. (2009). Islamic religiosity, subjective well-being, and health. *Mental Health, Religion & Culture*, *12*(1), 55-74.

Tessler, M. (2003). Arab and muslim political attitudes: stereotypes and evidence from survey research. *International Studies Perspectives*, 4, 175–180.

Weaver, A. J., Vane, A., & Flannelly, K. J. (2008). A review of research on Buddhism and health: 1980–2003. *Journal of health care chaplaincy*, *14*(2), 118-132.

Whitman, S. M. (2007). Pain and suffering as viewed by the Hindu religion. *The Journal of Pain*, *8*(8), 607-613.

Wig, N. N. (1999). Mental health and spiritual values. A view from the East. *International Review of Psychiatry*, *11*(2-3), 92-96.

Chapter 9

RELIGION, SPIRITUALITY AND THE END OF LIFE

Dying in our society has often become a protracted affair. 73% of deaths are among those who are at least 65 years old, and 24% are at least 85 years old. 40% of family members perceive that their loved one suffered unnecessarily in death. 10%-50% received care that violated their personal preferences (Puchalski, 2002). Death is a natural process. And yet, we medicalize death. We sterilize death with our technology and sterilize the deep questions that impending death stirs. 90% of patients would like to die at home if terminally ill. In our time, the opposite is true: 57% of deaths occur in the hospital, 37% are in nursing homes or other residencies (Puchalski 2002). Death is a natural process. Dying should also be a meaningful process. How do we make that happen? While there are many challenges and competing interests, our patients' spiritual values and religious traditions can be an important resource to balance the weight of modern medicine.

Palliative care, withdrawal of advanced life support, advanced care planning (i.e., living wills), euthanasia, and physician assisted suicide are challenging issues where one's religious and spiritual values have great influence in one's approach to decision making. Many religious groups offer guidelines and contribute to the public discourse around these issues – such as the National Conference of Catholic Bishops, the Unitarian Universality Assembly, and the Conservative Movement's Committee on Jewish Law and Standards (Daaleman and VandeCreek, 2000).

Patients facing end of life may be asking important questions about suffering, meaning, and love. Patients may be experiencing anger and regret about their condition. Self-blame, guilt, and denial may be strong emotional responses to a terminal diagnosis. Family members, similarly, may be wrestling with their own sense of loss and the complicated challenge of attending to the loved one's needs while grieving themselves. Physicians too may be struggling with their own secondary trauma in treating patients with terminal illness.

Religion and spirituality often serve as an attenuating influence in coping with terminal illness. In the first study to address spirituality, religiosity, and depression among the terminally ill, Nelson et al., (2002) studied a population of 162 patients with HIV and Cancer who were recruited from a palliative care facility who had life expectancy of less than 6 months. Spirituality, meaning, and sense of peace were inversely correlated with depression. Religiosity, however, did not have a significant impact with depression (Nelson et al., 2002). An important consideration in such studies is that the instruments used to study depression and spirituality are often quite similar. Questions of wellness and peace in the spirituality instrument are very similar to the items in the depression scale. Greater social support was associated with greater religiosity (rho = 0.18, $p < .05$), faith (rho = 0.24, $p < .05$), meaning (rho = 0.37, $p < .01$), and overall spirituality (rho-0.36, $p < .01$). Interestingly, the greater one's faith, the greater one's experience of pain (rho = 0.24, $p < .05$) (Nelson et al., 2002).

Perhaps no issue challenges religious belief than the issue of euthanasia and physician assisted suicide. In the Judeo-Christian tradition, one's life is not one's own, but belongs to God. "The Lord gave and the Lord taketh away." (Job 1:21) Thus, suicide is akin to stealing your life from God who is the arbiter of life and death. Several studies have shown that religious belief influences physicians' approach to euthanasia. Oncologists with high or moderate levels of religious belief were less likely to perform euthanasia or physician-assisted suicide than those with no religious belief (Emanuel et al., 1998). This study was echoed by Meier who showed that those physicians with no religious affiliation were more likely to provide assistance with a patient request for physician-assisted suicide (Meier et al., 1998). A survey among physicians, nurses, and social-workers in New York City endorsed the same sentiment (Portenoy et al., 1997).

Religious and spiritual questions arise in death. Faith – and lack of faith – is often part of common parlance. Patients with advanced breast cancer have shown greater spiritual well-being and self-transcendence if able to maintain a sense of purpose or meaning in life (Coward 1989; Dow et al., 1996). Among the terminally ill, spirituality is associated with subjective well-being, and lower levels of anxiety and psychological distress (Kaczorowski 1989; Reed,

1987; Smith et al., 1993). Among the terminally ill, patients higher in spiritual well-being were less likely to desire a hastened death ($r = -0.52$, $p < .0001$), hopelessness $r = -0.68$, $p < .0001$), and suicidal ideation ($r = -0.41$, $p < .0001$). This finding was significant even after controlling for depression and other demographic variables (McClain, Rosenfeld, & Breitbart, 2003). While spiritual well-being has been strongly correlated with lower depression scores, belief in an afterlife has also been shown to reduce end-of-life despair, such as desire for death, hopelessness, and suicidal ideation (McClain-Jacobson et al., 2004).

Hospice

An important institution that models an integrated approach of religion and medicine is the Hospice movement. Founded in the 1960's as a religious movement to provide compassionate, spiritually centered care for the terminally ill, it has expanded into a world-wide movement (Daaleman, 2000). Much of its explicitly Christian mission has been nuanced to include people from all traditions and cultures. In its medieval origins, a hospice was a lodging for travelers run by a religious order. Its core mission was hospitality to people on a journey. The same core mission is present today – to provide hospitality and solace to those on their final journey (Daaleman 2000). The medical needs are met in the context of a spiritually attune institution. The Hospice movement does not assume that religious or psychosocial dimensions are secondary to medical interests. All currents come together for the comfort of the patient.

The Patient, The Family and the Healthcare Provider

Another important nuance to a patient's spirituality needs to be considered in care at the end of life: the nature of a person's faith. A strong belief in God does not confer comfort at the end of life. Among patients with HIV, Kaldjian et al., (1998) showed that fear of death was more likely among patients who believed that HIV was a punishment ($p = .01$) or felt guilty about having HIV ($p = .039$) and was less likely among those who read the Bible frequently ($p = .01$) or attended church regularly ($p = .015$) (Kaldjian, Jekel, & Friedland,

1998). Other papers have shown similar findings: the attitude of one's faith determines one's coping. Perceiving illness as divine punishment is correlated with increased anxiety and fear (Pargament et al., 1990).

The other challenging dimension to end of life care is the complicated milieu of the family. The patient's faith may be in discord with the family's, making for challenging conversation around end of life care decisions. The other variable that is not often found in the literature is this: a dying person's spirituality is in a state of flux. The atheist may be questioning the existence of God. The devout Methodist may be angry at the seeming injustice of bodily suffering. The very framework of peoples' lives is being re-examined. "What happens after death?" may have been an abstract question among friends. This question takes on new meaning if the person faces terminal cancer.

Supporting our patients, affirming questions, incorporating spiritual care with chaplains can be an important process to dying. The spiritual journey may, in fact, be the most important aspect of a patient's dying.

Interventions are difficult to design given that it would be unethical to randomize patients to a "placebo" spiritual care arm. And so, we are left with the inferences derives from cohort studies. While this is unsatisfactory when running drug trials, the weight of evidence suggests something important: patients feel better when their spiritual needs are addressed, especially at the end of their lives.

Another important study among the terminally ill examined those with cancer who had greater than six months left to live and their desire for a hastened death. Interestingly, less than 2% of patients had a desire for an early death. The desire for an early death correlated positively with depression, hopelessness, and physical distress, and negatively with spiritual well-being, social support, and self-esteem. It was not associated with proximity to death (Rodin et al., 2007).

Addressing the spiritual care of the terminally ill is complicated. Physicians seem all too relieved to delegate the responsibility to the specialists such as chaplains or the patient's own clergy. In a large national survey, 80% of family physicians reported that they refer to pastoral care providers for issues around end-of-life care. (Daaleman & Frey, 1998). There are particular challenges for healthcare providers in addressing spiritual and religious issues of the terminally ill. We cannot but help face our own questions and worry about death and suffering. Can we be objective enough? Would we over medicate for pain, identifying too closely with the patient? Would we give up too soon? Too late? How do our own faith traditions impact our care of the patient? But is deferring the spiritual care an abrogation of a physician's responsibility? Is it merely a convenient excuse to refer spiritual questions to a professional clergy or chaplain?

In the same way that consultation with a specialist may yield a more nuanced, sophisticated intervention, this does not abrogate the physician from addressing the spiritual care of the patient. At no other place in healthcare are the currents of spirituality, technology, suffering, and patient uncertainty in greater confluence. Illnesses that require the greatest technological expertise also require the greatest emotional support. Questions of the most sophisticated scientific scope are matched only by the most dire spiritual ones.

Feelings of demoralization, isolation, anger, and grief are common among terminally ill patients. While these reactions are human, appropriate responses, processing one's death and coming to reconciliation is important for the patient's remaining days. Supporting a person in their grief and allowing for helpful spiritual care may lead to reconciliation and a "good death."

There is no more sacred moment in our craft as healthcare providers to be fully present to our patients in the moment of death. To sit at the bedside, engage with the patient and family takes spiritual strength and wisdom. We marshal our resources as best we can, seek help when needed, and re-discover our sacred purpose in our vocation: to relieve suffering.

REFERENCES

Coward, D. D. (1990). The lived experience of self-transcendence in women with advanced breast cancer. *Nursing Science Quarterly*, *3*(4), 162-169.

Daaleman, T. P., & Frey, B. (1998). Prevalence and patterns of physician referral to clergy and pastoral care providers. *ArcHIVes of Family Medicine*, *7*(6), 548.

Daaleman, T. P., & VandeCreek, L. (2000). Placing religion and spirituality in end-of-life care. *Journal of the American Medical Association*, *284*(19), 2514-2517.

Dow, K. H., Ferrell, B. R., Leigh, S., Ly, J., & Gulasekaram, P. (1996). An evaluation of the quality of life among long-term survivors of breast cancer. *Breast cancer research and treatment*, *39*(3), 261-273.

Emanuel, E. J., Daniels, E. R., Fairclough, D. L., & Clarridge, B. R. (1998). The practice of euthanasia and physician-assisted suicide in the United States: adherence to proposed safeguards and effects on physicians. *Journal of the American Medical Association*, *280*(6), 507-513.

Kaczorowski, J. M. (1989). Spiritual well-being and anxiety in adults diagnosed with cancer. *Hospice Journal*, 5:105-116.

Kaldjian, L. C., Jekel, J. F., & Friedland, G. (1998). End-of-life decisions in HIV-positive patients: the role of spiritual beliefs. *Aids*, *12*(1), 103-107.

McClain, C. S., Rosenfeld, B., & Breitbart, W. (2003). Effect of spiritual well-being on end-of-life despair in terminally-ill cancer patients. *The Lancet*, *361*(9369), 1603-1607.

McClain-Jacobson, C., Rosenfeld, B., Kosinski, A., Pessin, H., Cimino, J. E., & Breitbart, W. (2004). Belief in an afterlife, spiritual well-being and end-of-life despair in patients with advanced cancer. *General hospital psychiatry*, *26*(6), 484-486.

Meier, D. E., Emmons, C. A., Wallenstein, S., Quill, T., Morrison, R. S., & Cassel, C. K. (1998). A national survey of physician-assisted suicide and euthanasia in the United States. *New England Journal of Medicine*, *338*(17), 1193-1201.

Nelson, C. J., Rosenfeld, B., Breitbart, W., & Galietta, M. (2002). Spirituality, religion, and depression in the terminally ill. *Psychosomatics*, *43*(3), 213-220.

Pargament, K. I., Ensing, D. S., Falgout, K., Olsen, H., Reilly, B., Van Haitsma, K., & Warren, R. (1990). God help me:(I): Religious coping efforts as predictors of the outcomes to significant negative life events. *American journal of community psychology*, *18*(6), 793-824.

Portenoy, R. K., Coyle, N., Kash, K. M., Brescia, F., Scanlon, C., O'Hare, D., ... & Foley, K. M. (1997). Determinants of the Willingness to Endorse Assisted Suicide: A Survey of Physicians, Nurses, and Social Workers. *Psychosomatics*, *38*(3), 277-287.

Puchalski, C. M. (2002). Spirituality and end-of-life care: a time for listening and caring. *Journal of palliative medicine*, *5*(2), 289-294.

Reed, P. G. (1987). Spirituality and well-being in terminally ill hospitalized adults. *Research in nursing & health*, *10*(5), 335-344.

Rodin, G., Zimmermann, C., Rydall, A., Jones, J., Shepherd, F. A., Moore, M., ... & Gagliese, L. (2007). The desire for hastened death in patients with metastatic cancer. *Journal of pain and symptom management*, *33*(6), 661-675.

Smith, E. D., Stefanek, M. E., Joseph, M. V., Verdieck, M. J., Zabora, J. R., & Fetting, J. H. (1994). Spiritual awareness, personal perspective on death, and psychosocial distress among cancer patients: An initial investigation. *Journal of Psychosocial Oncology*, *11*(3), 89-103.

Chapter 10

RELIGION, SPIRITUALITY AND PSYCHOSIS

In the great debate between religion and medicine, perhaps there is no more complicated issue than psychosis, hallucinations, and other similar mental disorders. The church has had a complicated relationship with mystics – at times lauding them and other times vilifying them. St. Theresa of Avila had visions of the torments of hell. Hildegard of Bingen had visions of “viriditas” – the divine “green-ness” of the world. Both had a complicated relationship with the church during their lifetime. Demonic possession has been attributed to mental illness and epilepsy since before medieval times (Kemp & Williams, 1987). And yet, even in modern times, among patients who self identify as being religious, demon possession or influence by evil spirits was the explanation for 56% of self-described religious patients with schizophrenia, 48% in patients with anxiety disorders, 37% in those with personality disorders and 23% in adjustment disorders (Pfeifer 1999).

Sigmund Freud has classified religion as an illusion and neurosis that can be overcome through maturation, and a mass-delusion or a psychotic defense against reality (Freud 1934). Freud also believed that modern psychological theories would substitute for the old world religious beliefs (Freud 1930). Other historical leaders in psychiatry – notably Emil Karaepelin and Kurt Schneider - considered religion to be the cause of their patients’ psychosis. Phillipe Pinel affirmed this position and believed that patients should be deprived of their symbols and practice of their religion and instead taught philosophical and historical knowledge (Mandel, 1980).

In 2000, Mark Salzman published *Lying Awake* (Salzman, 2000). The story tells of a nun who, after years of spiritual drought, is gifted with intense mystical visions, followed by debilitating headaches. When she consults with a neurologist, he diagnoses a temporal lobe seizure disorder. The nun is faced with a difficult decision: take medications to treat her "disorder" or continue these debilitating visions. Her mystical experiences gave her a view into God's plan for the world, but their increasingly debilitating intensity threatened her ability to function in daily life. Salzman's work of fiction captures the tension between the church and modern medicine. What is a "legitimate" mystical vision? What is a pathological hallucination? How do you tell the difference?

Modern medicine has been less than understanding towards those claiming mystical visions. Indeed, religion's claim for legitimacy has led to great critique by modern science (Horton, 1974). In 1976, the Group for the Advancement of Psychiatry wrote that religion is a "borderline psychosis… a regression, an escape, a projection upon the world of a primitive infantile state." (Group for the Advancement of Psychiatry, 1976) Elsewhere, religion has been described as "a psychotic episode" (Horton, 1974) and "temporal lobe dysfunction (Mandel, 1980).

There is a biological model to describe psychosis and religious sentiment. Temporal lobe epilepsy and religious or paranormal experiences has long been recognized (Slater & Beard, 1963). The "limbic marker hypothesis" locates psychosis and religious belief along the same pathways in the limbic system (Saver & Rabin, 1997). The limbic system processes emotions and is thought to be a more instinctive pathway. This system produces perceptions of self-importance, harmonious feelings, and profound joy. These emotions overlap with religious sentiment and pathological delusion. The difference, psychologists state, is only a matter of degree.

Similarly, the reptilian amygdala has been implicated in the formation of delusional beliefs. The amygdala is responsible for processing emotional reactions, memories, and decision-making. Amygdala "lability" has been implicated in attaching greater significance to mundane events, amplifying their significance and leading to pathological belief (Persinger, 2001). The problem with this biological model for psychosis is manifold. Locating the structures responsible for housing the experiences is like giving the address for a person's home. Everyone has an amygdala that locates certain aspects of our experience. Because delusions and religious belief are processed through the same pathway does not automatically infer that religious belief is pathological. All experiences are processed through the amygdala and the limbic system – even normal ones. We cannot infer pathology simply because the same structures are used for pathological and normal experiences alike.

What is the church's divine gift can be medicine's pathology. In the Diagnostic and Statistical Manual of Mental Disorders, 4th edition (DSM-IV), a new diagnostic category was created, "religious and spiritual problem." (Turner et al., 1995) This serves a twofold, contradictory purpose. On the one hand, there is a defined, new area of clinical focus with a broad definition that can be separated from other pathological experiences. Providers can assess these religious and spiritual issues without pigeon-holing them into another, less accurate diagnosis. Such examples of this include a loss of faith, spiritual conflicts that arise from transcendental matters, or mystical experiences triggered by meditative practices (Lukoff, Lu, & Turner, 1992).

Lukoff et al., (1992) describe how some patients may experience mystical feelings of unity, alterations in time perception, loss of ego due to meditative practices, or even out of body experiences. These experiences may be categorized as "religious or spiritual problems" or even as true psychosis. And yet, these symptoms do not present serious psychological difficulties. And among some patients, they are adaptive responses to life experiences. On the other hand, religiousness and spirituality now becomes a diagnosable condition. This implies pathology where there might not be any.

Religious delusions can be differentiated from religious belief based on three consensus criteria: (1) the patient's self description of the experience is recognizable as a form of delusion, (2) other recognizable symptoms of mental illness are present in other areas of the individual's life (i.e., delusions, hallucinations, mood or thought disorder) and (3) the lifestyle, behavior and direction of the individual's goals after the religious experience are consistent with the history of a mental disorder rather than with a personally enriching life experience (Sims, 2009). Both psychosis and religious revelation are altered states of consciousness. The difference between the two is the capacity for the patient to differentiate between revelation and reality. Patients with psychosis are unable to tell the difference (Clarke 2001).

Grof & Grof (1989) posit a model to differentiate spiritual and religious problems and true psychosis. Spiritual insight is usually gradual, the product of study, reflection, and medication. Changes occur over time, are usually pleasant, and reinforce a positive attitude. Also, inner experience and external reality are well-differentiated: the mystic knows the difference between a spiritual experience and the world (Groff & Grof, 1989). Religious experiences connected to mental disorders are usually intense and abrupt, generate unpleasant sensations, and invoke confusion around the difference between experience and external reality (Grof & Grof, 1989). The other aspect to differentiate between religious emergence and religious psychosis is that true psychosis does not occur in isolation. Almost always, there are other aspects of disorganized thinking, paranoia, aggressiveness, or other history of psychiatric illness (Grof & Grof, 1989).

Menezes & Moreira-Aleida (2009) suggest a revision of the criteria to differentiate between spiritual experiences and mental disorders. They suggest that the following criteria would indicate that a religious experience would not be pathological:

- Absence of psychological suffering: the individual does not feel disturbed due to the experience he or she is having.
- Absence of social and occupational impediments: the experience does not compromise the individual's relationships and activities.
- The experience has a short duration and happens occasionally: it does not have an invasive character in consciousness and in the individual's daily activities.
- There is a critical attitude about the experience: the capacity to perceive the unusual nature of the experience is preserved.
- Compatibility of the experience with some religious tradition: the individual's experience may be understood within the concepts and practices of some established religious tradition.
- Absence of psychiatric comorbidities: there are no other mental disorders or other symptoms suggestive of mental disorders besides those related to spiritual experiences.
- Control over the experience: the individual is capable of directing his or her experience in the right time and place for its occurrence.
- Life becomes more meaningful: the individual reaches a more comprehensive understanding of his or her own life.
- The individual is concerned with helping others: the expanded consciousness develops a deep link with other human beings.

The other complicated nuance to psychosis and religious belief is culture. The belief in demons and angels may have a strong cultural element or be a means of explaining undue influence – "the devil made me do it" – that does not have the pathologic intensity of a true psychosis. Religious people may have beliefs about demons, without those beliefs being defined as psychosis. Another intriguing angle is the question: does religious affiliation place one at risk for psychosis? This is difficult to answer. The few studies that have attempted this question have been inconclusive (Peters et al., 1999; Clark, 1980; Getz, Fleck, & Strakowski, 2001). Some studies have suggested an increased frequency but not severity of religiously oriented psychosis. The caveat interpreting these studies is that religious people, when they have psychotic breaks, may manifest that psychosis in the language of their religious culture.

Further complicating this question of psychosis and religious is experience is the recognition that hallucinatory experiences can be present among patients in the nonclinical population. As early as the 19th century, Sidgewick et al., (1894) interviewed 7,717 men and 7,599 women. 7.8% of the men and 12% of the women had at least one experience of hallucinations in their lives. This has been replicated in more recent studies, where prevalence of hallucinations has occurred in 7.8%-15% of otherwise normal people (West 1948, Tien 1991). These experiences can be relatively common. In one western European study that evaluated 13,057 individuals, 19.7% had hallucinations less than once a month, 6.4% of them reported having had hallucinations more than once a month, 2.7% once a week, and 2.4% more than once a week (Ohayon 2000). In short, the general population has had or regularly has some form of auditory or visual hallucinations. The claims of modern medicine that hallucinations and delusions are pathological contain great truth. Another study showed that between 4-12% of the population in the United States will suffer from hallucinations and delusions. However, only 25% meet true criteria for psychosis. 75-90% of such non-pathological hallucinations are transitory and do not present significant risks to the people who experience them (Johns et al., 2002).

In contrast, people with schizophrenia may have delusions that do fit the definition of religious psychosis. This seems to carry across different cultures, but with varying degrees. The prevalence of religious delusions among patients with schizophrenia varies across different countries – 14-36% in the USA, 21% in Germany, 15% in Brazil, 7% in Japan, 6% in Pakistan (Applebaum, Robbins, & Roth 1999; Dantas, Pavarin, & Dalgalarrondo, 1999; Farr & Howe, 1932; Tateyama et al., 1993; Stompe et al., 1999). In another case series, 24% of hospitalized patients with schizophrenia had religious delusions (Siddle et al., 2002).

But is religiosity helpful for our patients suffering from psychosis? The data is equivocal. Among 115 patients in Switzerland, 85% consider religion to be important to their lives, and gave hope to 71%, but desperation to 14% (Mohr et al., 2006). At a 3 year follow up, 63% maintained their religious commitment. 20% reporting a positive changes to their lives, and 17% reporting negative changes to their lives. (Mohr et al., 2010). And yet, an interesting study among 323 schizophrenic patients in India noted improvement in symptoms with an increase in the patients' religious activities (Verghese et al., 1989). Religious involvement, it seems, can be a solution for some and a burden to others. Parsing who would benefit can be difficult and few studies have elucidated this.

TREATMENT

There can be synergy between religious and allopathic treatment strategies (Hale & Pnninti, 1994). In one ongoing study, more than half of the schizophrenic outpatients use spirituality on a large scale to cope with ongoing stress. One patient said, "Jesus is my only shield, I ask Him to help me in my daily activities, I feel that I am not alone. He shows me the way." (Mohr & Huguelet, 2004) The stakes for treating patients with psychosis is high. Suicide is as much as 10% among patients suffering from schizophrenia, and as many as 40% attempt suicide. Religion may be the one attenuating influence against suicide (Murphy, 2000). One patient with schizophrenia stated, "I don't know why I suffer from deep anxiety and hallucinations, the psychiatrist told me it was nerves, and the pastor and the members of my church pray for me to be delivered from bad things in the name of Jesus… it is God who gives wisdom to psychiatrist for medication, I pray for caregivers, I put my hope in God and I take my medication." (Mohr& Huguelet, 2004) Another patient said, "I don't know if what I see are the spirits of the dead or if I am crazy, so I have to learn more about spirituality and go on with psychiatric treatment" (Mohr& Huguelet, 2004).

Religious belief among patients suffering from schizophrenia is complex. One patient from Mohr and Huguelet's (2004) series states, "I believed I was possessed by demons, I'd go to an exorcist priest, he taught me the gospel and he case out the demons, he encouraged me to go to the psychiatrist. Now I believe half is schizophrenia, half is demonic possession, so I go on with the priest and I take half of my medication." Many religions disapprove of alcohol or drugs. (Kendler et al., 2003, Booth & Martin, 1998) Also, religious commitment has been associated with lower suicide attempts and suicidal deaths (Koenig, Larson, & Larson, 2001). In Mohr's qualitative study, one of their patients stated, "Even in the lowest moments of my life, I forbid myself suicide because of my religious background." Another patient stated, "God delivered me from smoking" (Mohr & Huguelet, 2004).

In the same way, religious belief can play into one's delusions. The desire to enjoy the afterlife, go to heaven, unite with God can all compel a person to consider suicide. Also, the strong normative culture of some religious communities may exclude those with mental illness. This effect may be overt: the community might shun a person with schizophrenia. One of Mohr's patients shared, "I am angry with some members of my community because I have not found any help at the human level, they moralized without knowing what I felt deep inside me" (Mohr& Huguelet, 2004).

Similarly, a patient with schizophrenia may believe they are unworthy, unwelcome, or too much of a sinner to participate in the community life. From Mohr & Huguelet's study (2004), a patient shared, "I went to the spirit center for 10 years, I had all my friends there. Once I smoked hashish and I went there drunk. They were amazed and I couldn't go again because they forbid drinking and smoking.... I don't know what I believe in anymore, I don't know who is right, the spirits, the Buddhists, the Christians, I am spiritually lost."

Menezes & Moreira-Almeida (2010) suggests that the study of religiosity and psychosis is underexplored. He suggests two broad themes that merit further investigation. First, religiosity should be evaluated in its impact upon patients with psychoses. Second, further work needs to elucidate the difference between spiritual experience and true psychosis. The interplay between mystical, religious experiences and psychosis is complex, should not be overgeneralized, and are fraught with cultural and historical interpretations that make understanding this interplay difficult.

The area of schizophrenia and psychosis can be problematic for clergy and healthcare providers alike. Schizophrenic patients can have religious delusions, but that does not mean that religion, in itself, is delusional. Religious belief can stabilize and comfort a patient or further convict them of their sinfulness and brokenness. Religious communities can provide support or further exclude and harm. Above all, religion is relevant to the lives of patients suffering from psychosis. Providers should be tolerant of patients' beliefs. Religion is not merely a continuum of psychosis – a healthy, milder form of psychosis versus a more dense severe experience. Religion is categorically different – with internal beliefs and extrinsic practices. And yet, the uncomfortable truth for apologists is simply this: religious belief and delusion can look very similar. What Freud and other skeptics said has the ring of truth. And yet, how we interpret the data usually is a reflection of our bias. Not all hallucinations are visions. People with psychosis can be religious, but it is not their religion that makes them psychotic. Some without schizophrenia will have visions that are not pathological. Being aware of these subtleties, and encouraging a balanced treatment plan when appropriate is key for the healthcare provider. The challenge, then, for providers – apologists and skeptics alike – is to consider the individual patient and how their belief connects with other aspects of their health and wellness.

References

Appelbaum, P. S., Robbins, P. C., & Roth, L. H. (1999). Dimensional approach to delusions: comparison across types and diagnoses. *American Journal of Psychiatry*.

Booth, J., & Martin, J. E. (1998). Spiritual and religious factors in substance use, dependence, and recovery. In: Koenig HG, ed. *Handbook of religion and mental health*. San Diego: Academic Press, 175–99.

Clark, R. A. (1980). Religious delusions among Jews. *American journal of psychotherapy*, 34, 62-71.

Clarke, I. (2010). Psychosis and spirituality: The discontinuity model. *Psychosis and Spirituality: Consolidating the New Paradigm, Second Edition*, 101-114.

Dantas, C. D. R., Pavarin, L. B., & Dalgalarrondo, P. (1999). Symptoms of religious content on psychiatric patients. *Revista Brasileira de Psiquiatria, 21*(3), 158-164.

Farr, C. B., & Howe, R. L. (1932). The influence of religious ideas on the etiology, symptomatology and prognosis of the psychoses: with special reference to social factors. *American Journal of Psychiatry*, *88*(5), 845-865.

Freud S. (1930). Civilization and its Discontents. London: Leonard & Virginia Woolf at the Hogarth Press.

Freud S. (1934). The Future of an Illusion. London: L. & Virginia Woolf at the Hogarth Press and the Institute of Psycho-analysis.

Getz, G. E., Fleck, D. E., & Strakowski, S. M. (2001). Frequency and severity of religious delusions in Christian patients with psychosis. *Psychiatry Research*, *103*(1), 87-91.

Grof, C., & Grof, S. (1991). The stormy search for the self: A guide to personal growth through transformational crises. *Los Angeles, California: JP Tarcher*.

Group For The Advancement Of Psychiatry. (1976). *Mysticism: Spiritual Quest or Psychic Disorder?* Group for the Advancement of Psychiatry, New York.

Hale, A. S., & Pinninti, N. R. (1994). Exorcism-resistant ghost possession treated with clopenthixol. *The British Journal of Psychiatry*, 165, 386-8.

Horton, P. C. (1974). The Mystical Experience: Substance of an Illusion, *American Psychoanalytic Association Journal* 22:(2): 364-380.

Johns, L. C., Nazroo, J. Y., Bebbington, P., & Kuipers, E. (2002). Occurrence of hallucinatory experiences in a community sample and ethnic variations. *The British Journal of Psychiatry*, *180*(2), 174-178.

Kemp, S., & Williams, K. (1987). Demonic possession and mental disorder in medieval and early modern Europe. *Psychological medicine*, *17*(01), 21-29.

Kendler, K. S., Liu, X. Q., Gardner, C. O., McCullough, M. E., Larson, D., & Prescott, C. A. (2003). Dimensions of religiosity and their relationship to lifetime psychiatric and substance use disorders. *American journal of psychiatry*, *160*(3), 496-503.

Koenig, H. G., Larson, D. B., & Larson, S. S. (2001). Religion and coping with serious medical illness. *Annals of Pharmacotherapy*, *35*(3), 352-359.

Lukoff, D., Lu, F., & Turner, R. (1992). Toward a more culturally sensitive DSM-IV: Psychoreligious and psychospiritual problems. *The Journal of nervous and mental disease*, *180*(11), 673-682.

Mandel, A. J., (1980). Towards a psychobiology of transcendence: God in the brain. In: "The Psychobiology of Consciousness," J. M. Davidson & R. J. Davidson (eds), Plenum, New York, pp 39-464.

Menezes Jr, A. D., & Moreira-Almeida, A. (2009). Differential diagnosis between spiritual experiences and mental disorders of religious content. *ArcHIVes of Clinical Psychiatry (São Paulo)*, *36*(2), 75-82.

Menezes Jr, A., & Moreira-Almeida, A. (2010). Religion, spirituality, and psychosis. *Current psychiatry reports*, *12*(3), 174-179.

Mohr, S., Borras, L., Rieben, I., Betrisey, C., Gillieron, C., Brandt, P. Y., ... & Huguelet, P. (2010). Evolution of spirituality and religiousness in chronic schizophrenia or schizo-affective disorders: a 3-years follow-up study. *Social psychiatry and psychiatric epidemiology*, *45*(11), 1095-1103.

Mohr, S., Brandt, P. Y., Borras, L., Gilliéron, C., & Huguelet, P. (2006). Toward an integration of spirituality and religiousness into the psychosocial dimension of schizophrenia. *American Journal of Psychiatry*. 163, 1952-1959.

Mohr, S. M., & Huguelet, P. (2004). Spirituality and religious practices among people suffering from schizophrenia in ambulatory care in Geneva. *European Psychiatry*, 19, 93S-93S.

Murphy, M. A. (2000). Coping with the spiritual meaning of psychosis. *Psychiatric Rehabilitation Journal, 24*(2), 179-83.

Ohayon, M. M. (2000). Prevalence of hallucinations and their pathological associations in the general population. *Psychiatry research, 97*(2), 153-164.

Persinger, M. A. (2001). The neuropsychiatry of paranormal experiences. *The Journal of neuropsychiatry and clinical neurosciences*, 13, 515-524.

Peters, E., Day, S., McKenna, J., & Orbach, G. (1999). Delusional ideation in religious and psychotic populations. *British Journal of Clinical Psychology, 38*(1), 83-96.

Pfeifer, S. (1999). Demonic attributions in nondelusional disorders. *Psychopathology, 32*(5), 252-259.

Salzman, M. (2000). *Lying awake*. New York: Alfred A. Knopf.

Saver, J. L., & Rabin, J. (1997). The neural substrates of religious experience. *The neuropsychiatry of limbic and subcortical disorders*, 195-207.

Sidgwick, H., Johnson, A., Myers, F. W., Podmore, F., & Sidgwick, E. M. (1894). Report on the Census of Hallucinations. In *Proceedings of the society for psychical research*, 10(26), 25-394.

Sims, A. (2009). *Is Faith Delusion?: Why religion is good for your health.* London: Bloomsbury Academic.

Siddle, R., Haddock, G., Tarrier, N., & Faragher, E. B. (2002). Religious delusions in patients admitted to hospital with schizophrenia. *Social psychiatry and psychiatric epidemiology, 37*(3), 130-138.

Slater, E., & Beard, A. W. (1963). The schizophrenia-like psychoses of epilepsy. *The British Journal of Psychiatry, 109*(458), 95-112.

Stompe, T., Friedman, A., Ortwein, G., Strobl, R., Chaudhry, H. R., Najam, N., & Chaudhry, M. R. (1999). Comparison of delusions among schizophrenics in Austria and in Pakistan. *Psychopathology, 32*(5), 225-234.

Tateyama, M., Asai, M., Kamisada, M., Hashimoto, M., Bartels, M., & Heimann, H. (1993). Comparison of schizophrenic delusions between Japan and Germany. *Psychopathology, 26*(3-4), 151-158.

Tien, A. Y. (1991). Distribution of hallucinations in the population. *Social psychiatry and psychiatric epidemiology, 26*(6), 287-292.

Turner, R. P., Lukoff, D., Barnhouse, R. T., & Lu, F. G. (1995). A Culturally Sensitive Diagnostic Category in the DSM-IV. *The Journal of nervous and mental disease, 183*(7), 435-444.

Verghese, A., John, J. K., Rajkumar, S., Richard, J., Sethi, B. B., & Trivedi, J. K. (1989). Factors associated with the course and outcome of schizophrenia in India. Results of a two-year multicentre follow-up study. *The British Journal of Psychiatry*, *154*(4), 499-503.

West, D. J. (1948). A mass observation questionnaire on hallucinations. *Journal of the Society for Psychical Research*, *34*(644-645), 187-195.

Chapter 11

Interventional Prayer, Distance Healing and Other Tests of Faith

The minister announces from the pulpit, "Are there any requests for prayer?" A man stands, and shares that his sister has a lump in her breast and is going for more tests that week. An elderly woman raises her hand, "My grand-daughter just lost her job and is having trouble making ends meet." A young man asks that the church pray for peace in the Middle East. To the believer, prayer is the natural expression of faith. A believer prays precisely because of her belief that there is a higher power, and this higher power will entreat upon those prayers. A believer prays because she feels closer to God. She prays because of the deep-seated belief that those prayers will somehow make a difference in the world.

The whole Christian tradition is the story of unfolding prayer - the great monastic movements of the Middle Ages, the pietist revivals of the Reformation, and the spirit-filled American Great Awakenings. These great movements are, at their core, driven by a believer's renewed enthusiasm for prayer. There are luminous, mystical works that inform our Christian lives. St. John of the Cross, a Spanish mystic of the 16th century, wrote *Dark Night of the Soul*, which tells of the soul's journey to union with God (May, 2009). *The Way of a Pilgrim*, an anonymous work, tells of a layman who discovers the healing power of the Jesus Prayer, perhaps the greatest work of spirituality in the Russian Orthodox tradition (Bacovcin,, 1978). There is Brother Lawrence's simple, beautiful, *Practicing the Presence of God*, which demonstrates who to incorporate prayer into the mundane tasks of the day (Lawrence, 2007). There are many more. Billions of believers pray for healing, for peace, for prosperity, and on and on. Prayer is they way believers commune with God.

But does it work?

To the unbeliever, prayer is complete folly. How could prayer make a difference? There is no One listening. Interventional prayer, distant healing, laying on of hands and other sorts of directly-applied, religiously-oriented practices are perhaps the most controversial research field in religion and health. Believers believe, no matter what a trial shows. Skeptics will always be skeptical. What occurs in worship, in the hearts of believers, billions of times around the world either works or does not. It is the most inane practice or the most cost-effective.

To study prayer is fraught with controversy. What exactly are you studying? If one thinks of prayer as a drug, you must know what you are studying. There are questions around purity of the sample, how the drug is administered, and dose. Must one be a believer for a prayer to work? Does it matter? To what extent does one's faith play a role? What of the fervency of one's prayer? Is corporate prayer in worship enough?

The other dimension of interventional prayer is studying the work of God. This is where the "prayer as drug" metaphor breaks down. A drug does what it does to cause an effect in the body. The drug plugs into a cell's receptor, activates an enzyme, or mimics a biological process to cause an effect in the body. Prayer does not do this. Prayer entreats upon a third party – God – to act in the life of the subject.

What about the desired result? Praying for the healing of a sprained ankle seems different than praying for a cure from stage IV pancreatic cancer? Entreating God for victory on the battlefield seems vainglorious: your opponent is praying for the same thing. In his 1854 inaugural address, Abraham Lincoln famously said, "Both read the same Bible, and pray to the same God; and each invokes His aid against the other. It may seem strange that any men should dare to ask a just God's assistance in wringing their bread from the sweat of other men's faces; but let us judge not that we be not judged. The prayers of both could not be answered; that of neither has been answered fully" (Lincoln & Sebald, 1950).

There is the familiar temptation scene where Jesus is challenged by the devil in the book of Matthew (4:1-11). The devil takes Jesus to the top of the temple and challenges him, "If you are the Son of God, throw yourself down. For it is written, 'He will command his angels concerning you, and they will lift you up in their hands, so that you will not strike your foot against a stone.' " (Mathew 4:5-6) Jesus answers him from the book of Deuteronomy in the Old Testament, "It is also written, 'Do not put the Lord your God to the test.' " (Matthew 4:7) By studying interventional prayer is this precisely what we are doing: putting the Lord God to the test? Christians themselves will debate this issue. A prayer is not a pagan incantation. God is not summoned to do your bidding the way your butler responds to your bell. Even among believers the role of prayer is controversial. This sensitivity is further heightened when scientists engage this subject.

Perhaps the largest trial that studied interventional prayer was the MANTRA II trial (Krucoff et al., 2005). This study evaluated distant healing and "noetic therapies" – defined as healing practices not mediated by tangible elements – in patients about to undergo percutaneous coronary intervention. This randomized prospective trial enrolled 748 patients into four arms: standard care, interventional prayer, a "music-imagery-touch" (MIT) arm, and both MIT and interventional prayer. The combined primary endpoint was adverse cardiac event, 6-month re-admission rate, or death. Secondary endpoints were 6 month major cardiac event, readmission and 6 month mortality. There was no different in this combined primary endpoint. However, MIT at 6 months was lower than with no MIT therapy (hazard ratio 0.35, $p = 0.016$) (Krucoff et al., 2005).

Another famous study led by Herb Benson et al., (2006) was a multi-centered trial of more than 1,800 patients from six centers. They sought to answer the question: is it the prayer itself or the patient's certainty that they are receiving prayer a significant variable in a patient's recovery from coronary artery bypass graft. The study had three arms: one group (604 patients) received interventional prayer and were told they might receive it, another (597 patients) did not receive interventional prayer after being told they might receive it, the third group (601 patients) were told they were going to receive interventional prayer and did receive prayer (Benson et al., 2006). There were no differences across the three groups in their 30 day complication rate. Those certain of receiving prayer had a slightly higher rate of complications (59% vs 51%) but was not statistically significant (Benson et al., 2006).

Several studies have shown some positive effects. Byrd (1988) performed a double-blind trial on 393 patients in the coronary care unit. In the intervention arm, 3-7 intercessors prayed for the patient in the Christian tradition while the patient was in the hospital. Patients in the treatment arm required less ventilatory support and required less antibiotics and diuretics. To handle differences in patients, each was given a "severity score" as an outcome. Patients in the intervention arm had a lower severity score. However, there was no difference in mortality. A similar study by Harris et al., (1999) showed significant treatment effects for some global severity scores, but there was no difference in mortality.

Collipp, (1969) performed an interventional prayer trial on 18 patients with leukemia. The intervention arm received daily prayer for 15 months versus standard therapy. Patients in the control arm had a higher death rate, but the results were not statistically significant and there were some methodological issues: namely there was a small sample size of 16 patients and two of the patients in the control arm had a particularly deadly form of leukemia.

An important meta-analysis by Masters et al., (2006) looked at 14 well-designed interventional trials published in the literature. These studies all evaluated interventional prayer in a variety of populations: patients in a coronary care unit, suffering from leukemia, rheumatoid arthritis, alcohol treatment programs. The study concluded that there was no effect by the interventional prayer on the measured outcome. They conclude, "The most parsimonious statement to be made from this literature is that there is no scientifically discernable effect that differentiates the status of individuals who are the recipients of IP from those who are not." (Masters, Spielmans, & Goodson, 2006) They go on to state, "It should be pointed out that all of these studies suffer from a major and unsolvable methodological flaw, that is, receipt of prayer cannot be controlled and therefore it is impossible to know to what degree individuals in the control groups were actually the recipients of the 'intervention' from loved ones, family members, clergy, or others apart from the research intercessors" (Masters, Spielmans, & Goodson, 2006).

What can we derive from these intervention studies? Should interventional prayer be jettisoned as a therapeutic modality? Should providers tell our patients that the prayers of their family members do not make a difference? Given the impossibility of an adequate control arm (people will always be praying for their loved ones), there will be no ability for evidence-based medicine to answer that question. It is a bold move that modern science even to attempt to answer this question of interventional prayer. I concur with Masters: it makes little sense to continue studying this area. I also believe that believers will always believe – even if presented with evidence to the contrary. Skeptics will always be skeptical – even if presented with overwhelming evidence. In the television series, Star Trek, the fiery doctor McCoy fired to his intrepid colleague and friendly rival, "Spock, sometimes you can't think your way to the truth. Sometimes, you must love your way to the truth." Indeed, I am not sure if an adequately designed intervention trial will ever be performed. And, even with significant "p values," the skeptic will always find something to critique. And even if the study is not significant, the believer will continue to believe.

REFERENCES

Bacovcin, H. (1978). The Way of a Pilgrim, And, the Pilgrim Continues His Way: A New Translation. New York: An Image Book, Doubleday Publishing.

Benson, H., Dusek, J. A., Sherwood, J. B., Lam, P., Bethea, C. F., Carpenter, W., ... & Drumel, D. (2006). Study of the Therapeutic Effects of Intercessory Prayer (STEP) in cardiac bypass patients: a multicenter randomized trial of uncertainty and certainty of receiving intercessory prayer. *American heart journal,* 151(4), 934-942.

Byrd, R. C. (1988). Positive therapeutic effects of intercessory prayer in a coronary care unit population. *Southern medical journal*, 81(7), 826-829.

Collipp, P. J. (1969). The efficacy of prayer: a triple-blind study. *Medical times*, 97(5), 201-204.

Harris, W. S., Gowda, M., Kolb, J. W., Strychacz, C. P., Vacek, J. L., Jones, P. G., ... & McCallister, B. D. (1999). A randomized, controlled trial of the effects of remote, intercessory prayer on outcomes in patients admitted to the coronary care unit. *ArcHIVes of Internal medicine*, 159(19), 2273-2278.

Krucoff, M. W., Crater, S. W., Gallup, D., Blankenship, J. C., Cuffe, M., Guarneri, M., ... & Pichard, A. (2005). Music, imagery, touch, and prayer as adjuncts to interventional cardiac care: the Monitoring and Actualisation of Noetic Trainings (MANTRA) II randomised study. *The Lancet*, 366(9481), 211-217.

Lawrence, B. (2007). Practicing the Presence of God: A Modernized Christian Classic. Brewster, MA: Paraclete Press.

Lincoln, A., & Sebald, H. (1950). The Emancipation Proclamation. Washington DC: National ArcHIVes and Records Service, General Services Administration.

Masters, K. S., Spielmans, G. I., & Goodson, J. T. (2006). Are there demonstrable effects of distant intercessory prayer? A meta-analytic review. *Annals of Behavioral Medicine*, 32(1), 21-26.

May, G. G. (2009). The dark night of the soul. Grand Rapids, MI: Zondervan.

Chapter 12

THE PERSONAL JOURNEY

In August 2014, the New York Post reported that 2 interns committed suicide within 1 week of each other (Cusma & Rosenbaum, 2014; Velez & Cohen, 2014). They had just graduated from medical school. They were in their first months working as a physician. They had earned spots at prestigious residency programs. Their obituaries read of being personable, friendly, well-liked, with stellar credentials. They had made it to the top. Their future was bright. After many years of coursework, the grind of medical school, the stress of it all, they were finally doctors. Why, then, not three months into residency did two interns feel so depressed, so forsaken, that suicide was their best option? I have no doubt there were serious underlying psychiatric issues at play. I believe the programs were well run and met the requirements of the American Council on Graduate Medical Education (ACGME).

And yet, something terrible, tragic happened. Suicide? Really? Having two interns commit suicide a week apart in the same city makes us all think about the environment in which we trained, our present job, and what the future holds. Physicians-in-training are not alone. Physicians, in general, are more than twice as likely to commit suicide as the general population (Lindeman, 1996).

While there is much to bemoan around the external world of medicine, there is much that is beautiful and sacred about our craft. Once in the exam room, there is a patient and a doctor. One is trying to get well. The other is trying to help. There may be time pressures, insurance issues, and high expectations. And yet, our craft is a sacred one like no other. We treat the sick and suffering, one patient at a time. Our profession merges the intellect, the soul, and the body. We are challenged to be in balance, in touch, with what it means to live, to heal, and to die. We must know the science, and the evidence. Yet, we must speak the language of the patient and connect where they are.

This is a difficult calling. No wonder physicians suffer burnout. No wonder we cringe at the encroachments of insurance companies, administrators, and more paperwork. The prevalence of burnout is high among physicians. One comprehensive study among more than 3,000 physicians showed that 66% of emergency department physicians are burned out (Shanafelt et al., 2012). The prevalence of burnout for the average physician is 44%, far higher than the general population (Shanafelt et al., 2012). Interestingly, those physicians in the surgical subspecialties who are highly recompensed are some of the most burned out physicians (Shanafelt, 2012). Another study showed that emergency department physicians had the same satisfaction with life as those who were victims of abuse (Lloyd, Streiner, & Shannon, 1994). An important survey among 20,000 physicians by the Deloitte consulting group quantified the pessimism among the profession (Deloitte, 2013). 57% of physicians say that the practice of medicine is in jeopardy. Nearly three quarters say that the best and brightest may not consider a career in medicine. 62% believe that physicians will retire early; and 55% believe physicians will scale back hours (Deloitte, 2013).

Physicians cite the challenge of paperwork and encroachment on home life as the major stressors. From the Canadian Physician survey, a physician comment commented,

> "I believe that most physicians unconsciously contracted with society to pursue their profession to the utmost of their ability and energy, to keep up their skills, and do whatever was needed to promote patient care.... In return we expected respect, the equipment to do the job, and freedom from financial anxieties. All 3 of these expectations have been abrogated, yet we continue to fulfill our side of the contract in confusion, disbelief, and a sense of betrayal." (Sullivan & Buske, 1998)

This breach of social contract may manifest itself as a business-oriented model of care where the doctor-patient relationship is supplanted by a provider-consumer relationship. In an effort to reform healthcare, widen accessibility, address quality measures, perhaps the sacred trust between physicians and society has been annulled for a formal, contractual relationship. Have we lost a core principle at the expense of modernizing healthcare?

In an editorial, an Idaho physician well articulates the breach of sacred trust,

> "Physicians are denigrated with the same zeal that our predecessors were apotheosized. Amid this cacophony, it becomes ever more difficult to attend to our societal and personal sworn duty of caring for the ill and tending to the infirm. The routine intrusion of the non-physician on our educated decisions and the implications of dishonesty regarding our provision of care by the bureaucracy erodes our professional confidence and effaces the ancient numinosity of the physician-patient relationship… The decline of the professional class precedes the decay of the culture." (Wurster 1992)

In a Medscape Primary Care roundtable discussion, a physician stated, "Most interventions meant to improve burnout have treated it like a psychiatric illness, not a rational response to a badly led, dysfunctional healthcare system." (Centor et al. 2012) Burnout itself may be a marker of the larger, systemic challenges in healthcare. Perhaps the solution is not to address burnout as an isolated entity but rather a symptom of a widespread insidious problem. Address the system, and perhaps burnout will decrease.

What are we healthcare providers to do right now?

While many demographic variables are associated with burnout, several studies reveal practices that may have a protective effect against burnout. Weiner et al., (2001) surveyed 130 physicians to explore their own self-care practices. The six main positive practices were spending time with family and friends, religious or spiritual activities, intentional self-care activities, finding meaning in work, setting limits at work, and adopting a healthy philosophical outlook (Weiner 2001). Warde et al., (1999) survey 656 physicians and revealed that the presence of a supportive spouse and the ability to manage conflict were associated with higher marital and parental satisfaction scores.

Mindfulness, spirituality, and reclaiming one's purpose have also been posited as a potential strategy to cope with the stresses of physician work-life. (Remen, 2001; Epstein, 1999) In a promising pilot study, Shapiro et al., (2005) randomized physicians in an 8 week mindfulness course versus a control group. The course taught participants techniques in meditation, contemplation, and yoga. Pre- and post-test surveys showed satisfaction with life, increased compassion, and decreased burnout (Shapiro et al., 2005).

In a study among resident physicians, Doolittle et al., (2013) showed that higher spirituality scores correlated with lower emotional exhaustion and depersonalization and higher personal accomplishment. In particular, the domain of spirituality with the strongest impact was the expression of humility in personal interactions. Using the Hatch Spiritual Involvement and Beliefs

Scale (SIBS), variables that ask, "When I am ashamed of something I have done, I tell someone about it," "When I wrong someone, I make an effort to apologize," explore the importance of interpersonal relationships (Hatch et al., 1998). Residents who scored higher in the domain of humility had higher personal accomplishment and lower scores for emotional exhaustion and depersonalization (Doolittle, Windish, & Seelig, 2013).

Also, certain emotional coping strategies were associated with lower burnout scores: strategy planning, acceptance, and positive reframing. In contrast, certain emotional coping strategies correlated with higher burnout scores: venting, denial, and self-blaming (Doolittle, 2013). This study suggests that there are personality factors, beyond personal demographic characteristics or work culture, that influence burnout.

As healthcare providers we are steeped in the tradition of modern medicine. We have been acculturated by powerful traditions. We have sacrificed much to sit at the bedside. We make medical decisions based on the evidence and reason. This is tried and true formula born from the centuries, beginning with Aristotle, flourishing in the Renaissance, and coming to fruition in the Enlightenment. And yet, we also recognize that the iron rule of reason is lacking and the culture of medicine is sometimes lacking heart. How do we bring the two worlds of the heart and mind together? How do we model the very best of the data about religion and medicine? How do we shape the culture of medicine and sensitize this community to the ache of the soul? As we are at the pinnacle of reason and the evidence-based way, this is our challenge, the next chapter of medicine.

REFERENCES

Centor, R. M., Morrow, R. W., Poses, R. M., Vega, C. P. (2012 November 13). Doc burnout -- worse than other workers.' *Medscape Roundtable in Primary Care*, Retrieved on February 20th, 2013 from, www.medscape.com/viewarticle/774013.

Cusma, K., Rosenbaum, S. (2014 August 18). NYU medical grad jumps to his death from dorm roof. New York Post. Retrieved on February 5th, 2016 from http://nypost.com/2014/08/18/nyu-medical-grad-jumps-to-his-death-from-dorm-roof/.

Deloitte Center for Health Solutions. (2013). Survey of US Physicians – Physician perspectives about health care reform and the future of the medical profession. Retrieved on February 5th, 2015 from https://www2.deloitte.com/content/dam/Deloitte/us/Documents/life-sciences-health-care/us-lshc-deloitte-2013-physician-survey-10012014.pdf.

Doolittle, B. R., Windish, D. M., & Seelig, C. B. (2013). Burnout, coping, and spirituality among internal medicine resident physicians. *Journal of graduate medical education*, *5*(2), 257-261.

Epstein, R. M. (1999). Mindful practice. *Journal of the American Medical Association*, *282*(9), 833-839.

Hatch, R. L., Burg, M. A., Naberhaus, D. S., & Hellmich, L. K. (1998). The spiritual involvement and beliefs scale: Development and testing of a new instrument. *Journal of Family Practice*, *46*(6), 476-487.

Lindeman, S., Laara, E., Hakko, H., & Lonnqvist, J. (1996). A systematic review on gender-specific suicide mortality in medical doctors. *The British Journal of Psychiatry*, *168*(3), 274-279.

Lloyd, S., Streiner, D., & Shannon, S. (1994). Burnout, depression, life and job satisfaction among Canadian emergency physicians. *The Journal of emergency medicine*, *12*(4), 559-565.

Remen, R. N. (2001). Recapturing the soul of medicine. *Western Journal of Medicine*, *174*(1), 4.

Shanafelt, T. D., Boone, S., Tan, L., Dyrbye, L. N., Sotile, W., Satele, D., ... & Oreskovich, M. R. (2012). Burnout and satisfaction with work-life balance among US physicians relative to the general US population. *ArcHIVes of internal medicine*, *172*(18), 1377-1385.

Shapiro, S. L., Astin, J. A., Bishop, S. R., & Cordova, M. (2005). Mindfulness-based stress reduction for health care professionals: results from a randomized trial. *International Journal of Stress Management*, *12*(2), 164.

Sullivan, P., & Buske, L. (1998). Results from CMA's huge 1998 physician survey point to a dispirited profession. *Canadian Medical Association Journal*, *159*(5), 525-528.

Velez, N., Cohen, S. (2014 August 22). Medical intern plunges to death off tower in NYC. New York Post. Retrieved on February 5th, 2016 from http://nypost.com/2014/08/22/medical-intern-jumps-to-death-in-nyc/.

Warde, C. M., Moonesinghe, K., Allen, W., & Gelberg, L. (1999). Marital and parental satisfaction of married physicians with children. *Journal of general internal medicine*, *14*(3), 157-165.

Weiner, E. L., Swain, G. R., Wolf, B., & Gottlieb, M. (2001). A qualitative study of physicians' own wellness-promotion practices. *Western Journal of Medicine*, *174*(1), 19-23.

Wurster, C. F. (1992). The descendency of the educated class. *Western Journal of Medicine*, 156:438.

Chapter 13

FUTURE DIRECTIONS

Much has been accomplished in the field over the past 30 years. Research in this field is legitimate, attracts interest from the public and enjoys much support from many corners of the medical community. Many medical schools have specific programs in spirituality and medicine, where faculty have dedicated their careers to this study. In Harold Koenig's massive *Handbook on Religion and Health* (Koenig, King, & Carson, 2012). He surveys more than 1,200 studies and 400 reviews. He concludes, "In the majority of studies, religious involvement is correlated with well-being, happiness and life satisfaction; hope and optimism; purpose and meaning in life; higher self-esteem; better adaption to bereavement; greater social support and less loneliness; lower rates of depression and faster recovery from depression; lower rates of suicide and fewer positive attitudes towards suicide; less anxiety; less psychosis and fewer psychotic tendencies; lower rates of alcohol and drug use and abuse; less delinquency and criminal activity; greater marital stability and satisfaction." (Koenig, King, and Carson, 2012) Even the most ardent skeptic would have difficulty refuting such a substantial corpus of data.

And yet, there are many challenges. The vast majority of the research is observational where disparate variables are correlated together. Religiosity has been found to be helpful for a wide variety of conditions – from hip fractures to addiction. And yet, these studies are correlations only: a particular population is examined at a particular moment in time. Conclusions are drawn, but the caveat is always the same: correlation does not imply causation. For example, people who attend religious services are less depressed. And yet, if one suffers from severe depression, they may lack the psychomotor momentum to attend religious services. And so, is church attendance simply a marker of mental health? Sick people cannot make it to church, and so church attendees are healthier. Sick people cannot make it to the supermarket. But, we do not assume that shopping is protective against health. And yet, this standard refutation begins to ring hollow when the weight of the data is so compellingly positive. We are social animals who seek connection with others and with our world. We are intellectual creatures who thrive on thoughts and data. We are also soulful creatures who enjoy art, music, and poetry. Religion and spirituality is where these worlds intersect.

It is difficult for the healthcare provider to prescribe a dose. This is what we do after all: prescribe treatments for our patients. And so if the bulk of the data is observational, then the question to ask is: how much? What dose? What intensity? For example, does one need to achieve a threshold "dose" of church: once a month gets you no benefit, but twice a month is as good as every week?

What sort of religious involvement should we prescribe? Mindfulness exercises or traditional healing services? Is Bible study as good as a traditional service? Does one get the same effects from a church service on-line or via television compared to live attendance? Are there particular religious sects or denominations that have a stronger health benefit? The Adventists and Mormons have the best health profiles. Should we prescribe these? While this sounds facetious, it opens the question about what exactly providers should advise. Does everyone need a spiritual guide, a priest, a pastor, a rabbi, and an imam in the same way that one has a primary care physician? The answer is that, "It depends." It depends upon the patient, the disease, and the resources.

Role of the Chaplain and Pastor

In primary care, when our patients are complicated, we are quick to refer to the counselor, the social worker, and the care coordinator. We are ready to have the visiting nurse perform home safety assessments and medication checks. The Medical Home movement – where a team-based approach uses the skills of social workers, nurses, care coordinators, and others - goes a long way towards meeting the complex needs of our patients. More importantly, the Medical Home model delegates tasks to those more suitable to perform them: the referral coordinator, the patient navigator, etc. Given that so many of our patients' issues revolve around emotional and psychiatric burdens, is there a place for a religious figure in the medical home? Data on the role of the religious figure in the health care team is sparse. Does it make a difference? While the data on our patients' religious involvement demonstrates many advantages, the specific role of the religious figure in the health care team has only begun to be studied.

In a survey of 3,141 recently discharged patients, William et al., (2011) found that 41% of patients wished a discussion about their religious or spiritual concerns, yet only half reported actually having had such a discussion. Those patients who did have discussions related to their religious and spiritual concerns were more likely to rate the highest level of patient satisfaction in all categories (OR 1.4-2.2, 95% CI 1.1-3.0) (Williams et al., 2011). In a landmark study by Balboni et al., (2011), 339 patients with terminal cancer were asked about the spiritual and religious support received during their illness. Those who reported that their spiritual and religious needs were inadequately addressed were less likely to receive a week or more of hospice (54% vs 72.8%, $p = .01$) and were more likely to die in an intensive care unit (5.1% vs 1.0%, $p = 0.03$). End of life costs were higher when patients reported that their spiritual needs were inadequately supported ($4947 vs $2833, $p = .03$), particularly among minorities ($6533 vs 2276, $p = .02$) and high religious copers ($6344 vs $2431. P = .005) (Balboni et al., 2011). Patients with terminal illness, who received spiritual support from the medical team and pastoral care visits from chaplaincy had higher quality of life scores near death. Patients who used religious coping were also more likely to receive hospice (OR 4.93, 955 CI 1.64-14.80, $p = .004$) and less likely to receive aggressive care (OR 0.18, 95% CI, 0.04-0.79, $p = .02$) (Balboni, 2011). In another study that tapped the American Hospital Association survey database showed lower rates of hospital deaths ($B = .04$, $p < .05$) and higher rates of hospice enrollment ($B = .06$, $p < .001$) in hospitals that provided chaplain services compared to those hospitals that did not (Flannelly et al., 2012). In contrast, a multi-site longitudinal cohort study evaluated religious coping among patients with advanced cancer. 345 patients were assessed. Patients with positive religious coping were more likely to receive intensive life-prolonging care near death (OR 2.90, 95% CI, 1.07-7.89, $p = .04$) (Phelps et al., 2009).

Several important considerations need to be made. First, the gap between the chaplain and the medical team needs to be crossed. More integration is necessary for the improvement of our patients' care. This is most easily accomplished by inviting, insisting perhaps, that the chaplain be present at discharge conferences, care coordination meetings, or on medical rounds. The push-back on this plan, in my opinion, is from both the chaplains and the physicians. From the chaplains, there are simply not enough of them to go around to all the teams. The "congregation" for a thoughtful chaplain includes the staff as well as the patients. A chaplain colleague compared the hospital to a church where the steady "members" are the regular staff and the "visitors" are the patients. A chaplain presence integrated into the medical team serves the patient as well as providing support and care for the staff. While the one-on-one bedside interactions are the bedrock of the chaplaincy, as the healthcare system becomes more team-oriented, the chaplain needs to have a place at the table. From the physician-led teams, the presence of the chaplain would be one more voice that would slow down the already arduous task of patient care. Reviewing the labs, vitals, exam, considering the differential and crafting the plan of the day is already time-consuming, how would a chaplain add to that?

On the outpatient side, there are numerous barriers to inviting the religious figure into the care of the patient. Ministers are busy people. Their job contains a diverse skill set – public speaking, administration, personal counseling, and on and on. The pastoral visit is a key element in congregational care. As a pastor myself, a phone call from a physician would carry great weight in prioritizing my pastoral care visits. On the outpatient physician side, calling a patient's pastor requires disclosure agreement forms to be signed – one more task in an already busy day. And yet, the minister's presence in the care of a patient shows great promise. If the patient were getting emotional support from another skilled professional, might it make the healthcare provider visit more fruitful?

RELIGION AND FUTURE STUDY

Religion is complex – one part personal, one part communal, one part existential. Above all, religion is sacred. Religion cannot be reduced to a biological mechanism, a therapeutic tool, a dose to prescribe - despite modern medicine's best intentions to squeeze religion into an empirical framework. Religion is bigger than that. And yet, religion is not so sacred that we providers should not engage our patients' beliefs. Religion is too important to overlook. We providers need to be comfortable with our own spiritual identity, so that we can engage the question with our patients.

Thoughtful intervention trials are needed. Pharmaceutical companies spend billions developing drugs in careful double blind, case-controlled fashion. This has become the gold standard to legitimize a treatment. Should religion and spirituality be held to the same standard? Some would say yes. Attempts have been made to replicate this method in the realm of religion with equivocal conclusions. The challenge is that the “blind” part of the double blind trial. How can you control for religious involvement when so much of the population, in some way, expresses some religious involvement or spiritual attitude.

When religion works, there is nothing better – nothing more supportive, uplifting, or inspired. When religion does not work, there is nothing worse – nothing more violent, demeaning, judgmental, destructive, or harmful. A religious service might be the most intellectual and artistic experience in a person’s life – from the sermon to the hymn singing. Compared to secular methods of coping, religion may offer the most integrated perspective in an angst-ridden post-modern age. In a world of much clatter and “clever” YouTube videos, incessant list-serves, and reality television shows, religious life can be the crucial, sacred pause that gives perspective and hope in a noisy world.

For the most part, religious organizations get it right – as the data in this book has shown. And yet, there is always more to do – on the part of healthcare, religious organizations, and the individual. There are areas that are ripe for research. In particular, there are very few studies that evaluate religiosity and spirituality in a longitudinal fashion. Does the religious adolescent become a religious young adult? The evidence would say yes. And yet, how does religious coping change over time? Does the young parent seek religious and spiritual comfort differently than the elderly retiree? Nearly all studies are snapshots in time: cohort studies, convenience surveys, and qualitative interviews. But, what happens years later? Burnout is prevalent in the lives of physicians. Do people burnout from their religion? Who? How? Why? What happens to their health?

There are other ripe areas for research. There are almost no studies that address the religiosity and spirituality of gay, bisexual, and transgendered. These are the people that many religions reject out of hand. And yet, the tide is turning and many religious denominations have embraced same-gendered marriage. How do these sexual minorities perceive their spiritual lives in the face of institutional rejection? These are subtle, nuanced questions – especially in light of changing popular sentiment towards gays, lesbians, and the transgendered. Another important group are religious minorities and immigrants. Religion and culture are intertwined – especially among immigrant groups. How does religion impact mental and emotional health among Muslim immigrants? Buddhist families? Is religious dedication stronger among immigrant groups as a source of support and comfort? Does religious sentiment wane as immigrant groups assimilate into their host country? There is little data that explores this. Also, religion in America is changing. The second largest religious group (and fastest growing) are the "nones" – those who claim no religious affiliation. The "nones" account for 16-20% of the population (Pew, 2012). Are their lives completely devoid of spiritual questions or religious, ritualistic practices? Doubtful. Exploring this new emerging, evolving segment of the population is important.

Finally, there is a need for translation. Pierre Teilhard de Chardin, the French philosopher, Jesuit priest, and paleontologist, is credited with writing, "We are not human beings having a spiritual experience; we are spiritual beings having a human experience." Our intellectual, spiritual, and physical lives are inextricably women together. Perhaps it is our modern society that seeks to pick the tendrils apart. There is much work to be done to see the human being as a fully human, integrated being. Much progress has been made in the modern medical school curriculum. Is the Krebs cycle more important than the psychosocial history? As William Osler famously said, "The good physician treats the disease; the great physician treats the patient who has the disease." (Osler, 1909) This book is a humble attempt to move the conversation forward. Indeed, our very lives, and our patients' lives, may depend upon it.

There is ample evidence to suggest that religious involvement and spiritual practice are beneficial to one's health. Attendance at religious services and individual prayerful practices have shown repeated benefits to one's health. Religious people live longer, have less chronic disease, and suffer less depression (Koenig, King, & Carson, 2012). The question before healthcare providers: do our own lives model what the evidence suggests? Do we do what we tell our patients to do? Do we practice what we preach? Sorting out these questions for ourselves as providers is crucial to our professional happiness. Who wants to spend time with a cranky, over-worked doctor?

But what to do? The answer? Something. Almost anything. Real intervention studies are sparse. And yet, we can model successful endeavors. In 2009, Gretchen Rubin wrote the book, *The Happiness Project.* (Rubin, 2009) A Yale-trained lawyer, Rubin was feeling in a rut. She made a resolution to take on a new project each month of small steps to improve her overall happiness. One month was tidying her apartment 10 minutes a day – a small discipline which she credits for greatly improved overall life satisfaction. Another month, she tried out a personal trainer to incorporate exercise into her life. Another month, she worked on her marriage. The tone of her book was playful and good-humored. She appeals to those who are goal-oriented, those who like a checklist in their lives.

There are many other avenues to try. The point here is that *we must try something*. We must advocate to our patients to try something that fits their inclination, to explore their spiritual lives as we encourage them to eat right and exercise. We must do this for our patients - and for ourselves. Our patients need us at our best. The time of the "religiosity gap" – the dissonance between religion and medicine – is over. The benefits are too compelling. In an era of ever-increasing costs, ever louder critique of the medical system, religion and spiritual involvement shows great promise to be part of the solution. The time is now.

REFERENCES

Balboni, T., Balboni, M., Paulk, M. E., Phelps, A., Wright, A., Peteet, J., ... & Prigerson, H. (2011). Support of cancer patients' spiritual needs and associations with medical care costs at the end of life. *Cancer*, *117*(23), 5383-5391.

Flannelly, K. J., Emanuel, L. L., Handzo, G. F., Galek, K., Silton, N. R., & Carlson, M. (2012). A national study of chaplaincy services and end-of-life outcomes. *BMC palliative care*, *11*(1), 10.

Koenig, H., King, D., & Carson, V. B. (2012). *Handbook of religion and health*. Oxford, UK: Oxford university press.

Osler, W. (1909). *The principles and practice of medicine*. New York: Appleton and Company.

Pew Research Center, The Global Religious Landscape, December 18th, 2012, Retrieved on April 15th, 2015 from, http://www.pewforum.org/2012/12/18/global-religious-landscape-exec/.

Phelps, A. C., Maciejewski, P. K., Nilsson, M., Balboni, T. A., Wright, A. A., Paulk, M. E., ... & Prigerson, H. G. (2009). Religious coping and use of intensive life-prolonging care near death in patients with advanced cancer. *Journal of the American Medical Association*, *301*(11), 1140-1147.

Rubin's, G. (2009). *The happiness project*, New York: Harper Collins Publishers.

Williams, J. A., Meltzer, D., Arora, V., Chung, G., & Curlin, F. A. (2011). Attention to inpatients' religious and spiritual concerns: predictors and association with patient satisfaction. *Journal of General Internal Medicine*, *26*(11), 1265-1271.

ABOUT THE AUTHOR

Benjamin Doolittle is an Associate Professor of Internal Medicine and Pediatrics at the Yale School of Medicine. He joined the faculty in 2002 where he directs the Internal Medicine-Pediatrics residency program and serves as medical director of the faculty-resident clinic. He continues to serve the local church in a variety of capacities – supervised ministry mentor, pastor, and preacher. Ben is married to Christine and together they raise their two daughters with lots of help from Grandparents.

INDEX

C

D

E

F

G

H

I

J

K

L

M

N

O

P

Q

R

S

T

U

V

W

Y

Z